The Botany and Chemistry of Cannabis

THE BOTANY & CHEMISTRY OF CANNABIS

Proceedings of a Conference organized by The Institute for the Study of Drug Dependence at The Ciba Foundation 9-10 April 1969

Edited by:

C. R. B. JOYCE and

S. H. CURRY

*Department of Pharmacology and Therapeutics,
London Hospital Medical College*

1970

J. & A. CHURCHILL · LONDON

First Published 1970

International Standard Book Number
0.7000 14 79.9

Printed in Great Britain by
Spottiswoode, Ballantyne & Co. Ltd., London and Colchester

Contents

v

Participants

Dr. S. Agurell, Pharmaceutical Institute, University of Uppsala, Sweden.

Professor H. J. Bein, CIBA, CH 4000, Basle 7, Switzerland.

Dr. O. J. Braenden, United Nations Narcotics Laboratory, Palais des Nations, Geneva, Switzerland.

Professor L. Crombie, Department of Chemistry, University College, Cathays Park, Cardiff.

Dr. A. S. Curry, Forensic Science Laboratory, Home Office Central Research Establishment, Aldermaston, Reading, Berks.

Dr. S. H. Curry, Department of Pharmacology and Therapeutics, London Hospital Medical College, Turner Street, London E.1.

J. Dittert, Esq., International Narcotics Control Board, Geneva, Switzerland.

Professor J. W. Fairbairn, Department of Pharmacognosy, School of Pharmacy, Brunswick Square, London W.C.1.

Sir Harry Greenfield, International Narcotics Control Board, Geneva, Switzerland.

Dr. H. Halbach, World Health Organization, Geneva, Switzerland.

Dr. A. Haney, Department of Botany, 297 Morrill Hall, University of Illinois, Urbana, Ill. 61803, U.S.A.

Dr. C. R. B. Joyce, Department of Pharmacology and Therapeutics, London Hospital Medical College, London E.1.

Professor F. Korte, Institute of Organic Chemistry, Meckenheimer Allee 168, University of Bonn, 55 Bonn, W. Germany.

Professor Z. Krejčí, Department of Hygiene and Epidemiology, Palacký University, Oloumoc, Czechoslovakia.

Dr. V. Kuśević, United Nations Division of Narcotic Drugs, Palais des Nations, Geneva, Switzerland.

Dr. R. E. Lister, A. D. Little, Inc., Musselburgh, Scotland.

Professor R. Mechoulam, Laboratory of Natural Products, School of Pharmacy, Hebrew University, P.O.B. 517, Jerusalem.

Professor C. J. Miras, Department of Clinical Biochemistry, University of Athens, Greece.

Dr. A. Nordal, Pharmaceutical Institute, University of Oslo, Norway (P.O.B. 1068, Oslo 3).

Professor W. D. M. Paton, Department of Pharmacology, University of Oxford, South Parks Road, Oxford.

Dr. Th. Petrzilka, Laboratorium für organische Chemie, Eidgenössische Technische Hochschule, Universitätstrasse 6, 8006 Zürich, Switzerland.

Dr. R. K. Razdan, A. D. Little, Inc., Acorn Park, Cambridge, Mass. 02140, U.S.A.

Dr. R. Porter, CIBA Foundation, 41 Portland Place, London, W.1.

Dr. R. E. Schultes, Curator of Economic Botany and Executive Director, Harvard Botanical Museum, Oxford Street, Cambridge, Mass. 02138, U.S.A.

Dr. J. A. Scigliano, Center for Narcotic and Drug Abuse, National Institute of Mental Health, 5454 Wisconsin Avenue, Bethesda, Maryland 20015, U.S.A.

Dr. A. T. Shulgin, 1483 Shulgin Road, Lafayette, Cal. 94549, U.S.A.

Dr. W. T. Stearn, British Museum (Natural History), London, S.W.1.

Foreword

Sir Harry Greenfield, C.S.I., C.I.E.

Chairman, International Narcotics
Control Board, Geneva

This record of the first symposium organized by the Institute for the
Study of Drug Dependence is one step towards the vital task of
providing scientifically accurate material for those who wish to inform
themselves on the hazards of resorting to drugs which affect the central nervous system. As part of the Institute's broad programme
related to the various aspects of drug dependence, the Council hopes,
if its budget permits, to arrange a series of symposia covering the
whole field of these substances. Its choice of Cannabis as the first
subject of study was made for three reasons:

—because misuse of this substance has grown spectacularly in recent
  years and is still spreading;
—because it occupies a central position in the category of mind-
  affecting drugs; and
—because it figures prominently in the current world-wide debate
  on these drugs, and opinion on the risks attaching to its use
  ranges uncertainly between two extremes.

The purpose of this symposium was to establish botanical and
chemical specifications for materials used in pharmacological and
medical study, so as to permit comparison of results from different
research workers. This task has been well fulfilled by the impressive
combination of talent and experience which was assembled in the
group. Their findings will provide a firm basis for the wide range
of further studies which will now have to be made, if the challenge
presented by indulgence in cannabis is to be adequately met.

This indulgence is of course but one part of the phenomenon of
drug abuse, which is of special moment to all those who are concerned

with young people in the countries affected; whether they be parents, educationalists, members of the social services or of the medical or legal professions, or engaged in national or international controls over dangerous drugs.

The conscience of the world has been awakened to the grave dangers inherent in this phenomenon and much thought and expertise are being brought to bear on it by governmental and professional agencies in a number of countries. Such reinforcement is welcome because there is so much to be done and the need for accurate and detailed knowledge is urgent. Even in the matter of cannabis we are still only on the threshold of the area which requires to be explored.

Anyone who can claim real acquaintance with the question of drug abuse will agree that there is a vast amount to be learned before a satisfactory solution of this great social problem of our time can begin to be propounded, and that the search will have to be pursued in cooperation between all the disciplines which are involved.

The findings of this symposium on the botany and chemistry of cannabis and derivatives of substances obtained from it provide an essential foundation for future investigations by the Institute for the Study of Drug Dependence and other agencies of medical, psychiatric, behavioural and other aspects of cannabis consumption; and those who participate in these investigations will assuredly be grateful to the distinguished scientists who formed this symposium.

A special tribute of gratitude is due to the Ciba Foundation, which joined in sponsoring the symposium and generously provided the physical setting for it.

Introduction

C. R. B. Joyce and S. H. Curry

Drug dependence embraces diverse scientific disciplines, from
physical chemistry to social anthropology and makes overtures to
areas that are not scientific at all—to journalism, politics and international economics, for example. But this very breadth makes it difficult to develop comprehensive descriptions which are an essential
preamble to constructive social policies. Organizers of Symposia on
Drug Dependence have often optimistically sat chemists, psychologists,
pharmacologists and sociologists down together in the hope that
they will learn each others' languages and skills; but such hopes seem
in the event no less likely to increase misunderstandings than the
contrary.

For the first major public activity of the Institute for the Study
of Drug Dependence, therefore, the "hard" were deliberately separated from the "soft" scientists so that the former could reach as
much agreement as possible among themselves without being required to communicate with a much wider audience prematurely.
A second conference, planned to take place in 1971, will bring
together psychiatrists and other medical specialists, sociologists,
social psychologists and anthropologists; the way having been cleared
for them to discuss the employment of cannabis, its constituents
and their derivatives by the definitions and clarifications achieved
at the first meeting.

Pharmacology, more than any other subject, has one foot firmly
in each camp, and pharmacologists were therefore invited to the
present conference as they will be to the second. Some pharmacological reports and speculations in the present Proceedings thus make a
bridge to the next.

This record of the meeting differs in several ways from the proceedings as they actually occurred. The order of the papers has

been changed. The authors of some communications did not wish these to be published. The Discussions ranged back and forth between botany, chemistry and other matters, and have been severely edited and reshaped to fit the more formal structure of the book. Some sections of the formal contributions have also been modified to avoid overlapping or reference to certain matters outside the scope of the first conference. Most importantly, two additional contributions (those by Dr. Stearn and Professor Crombie) were invited after the meeting had ended, the need for them having become apparent meanwhile.

The Editors accept full responsibility for deficiencies of style or clarity in presentation. We are grateful that though the authors may have expressed themselves more elegantly at the time than the editors have made them appear to do, they will be content with the form that the work has taken. They have been particularly indulgent in the interests of rapid publication.

We are also extremely grateful to Dr. Hedy Kay for her invaluable work in checking formulae and translating some of the captions to the illustrations.

PART ONE
BOTANY

1 The Cannabis Plant: Botanical Characteristics

William T. Stearn

Despite much variation among individual plants of hemp (*Cannabis sativa* L.) in habit and size, the species is so distinct from all others that it can be recognized at all stages of growth by its botanical characters. These are accordingly set out below in language as non-technical as possible, for the use of persons with no botanical knowledge whose duties require them to identify *Cannabis*. The fibres of the stem produce the hemp used for canvas, ropes, etc., the glands of the female inflorescence the narcotic resin, the seeds an oil for paints; the seeds are also used as food for poultry and cage-birds.

Plants of *Cannabis sativa* (Fig. 1A) grow 1-5 m (3-15 ft.) high and are variously branched or even unbranched if crowded closely together; when bruised they have a distinctive somewhat unpleasant smell. A very rapid growing erect annual, *Cannabis sativa* is sown in Europe, as Rabelais said long ago, "at the first coming of the swallows and pulled out of the ground, when the cicadas begin to get hoarse", i.e. it completes its life-cycle within a few months. Seeds usually germinate within 3 to 7 days. The *seedlings* have two seed-leaves (cotyledons) slightly unequal in size, 1.0-1.6 cm (about ½ in.) long, mostly oblanceolate in shape (i.e. about 3 times as long as broad and broadest above the middle), narrowed to the base and rounded or blunt at the tip, with 3 main longitudinal veins, profusely sprinkled on the upper surface with minute hairs just visible under x10 magnification, each with a pustular or pearl-like base, hairless on the lower surface. The two seed-leaves are upheld by a relatively long stalk (hypocotyl) sometimes as much as 5 cm (2 in.) long. The first pair of true leaves arise on the stem about 2.5 cm (1 in.) or less above the seed-leaves; each leaf is distinctly stalked, with a narrowly elliptic blade shallowly saw-toothed (serrate) along the edge. The leaves

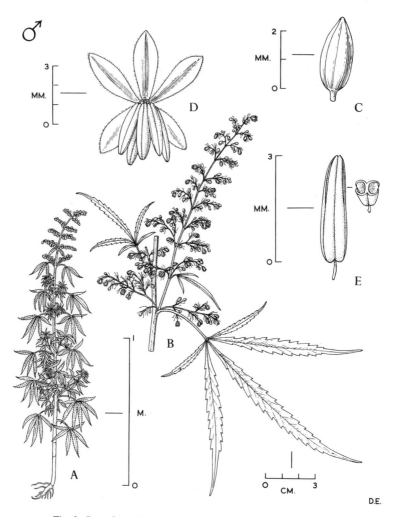

Fig. 1. Cannabis sativa; male plant. Primary specimen: W. J. Dress, No. 1135a in British Museum (Natural History), London.

of the second pair are much larger; they may be the same in shape as the first leaves or each may have a long stalk (petiole) with 3 leaflets radiating from its tip. Leaves of the third pair have 4 or 5 leaflets all radiating from the tip of the leaf-stalk and hence are described as digitate. Subsequent leaves higher on the stem may have

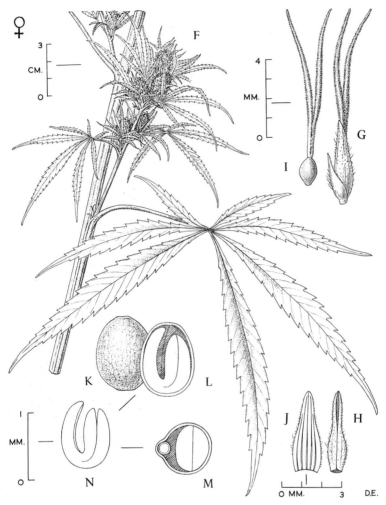

Fig. 2. Cannabis sativa; female plant. Primary specimen:
Mary F. Spencer, No. 887; fruit from Virginius H. Chase, No.
13005 in British Museum (Natural History), London.
Figs. 1 and 2 drawn by D. Erasmus.

as many as 11 leaflets and are arranged alternately (spirally) instead
of being paired.

   The *stem* (cf. Fig. 2F) is angular and sometimes hollow. It is
covered with minute hairs curved upwards and appearing as if pressed

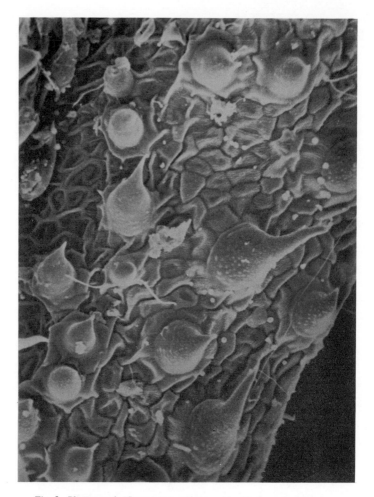

Fig. 3. Photograph (Stereoscan microscope) of hairs on upper surface of leaf of *Cannabis sativa*. Magnification x340. Photograph: Sims and Stearn, Electron Microscopy Unit, British Museum (Natural History), London.

against the stem. Similar hairs visible at x10 magnification occur on most parts of the plant. Each hair is formed from one cell; it narrows rapidly from a stout base to an acute tip; the base contains cystoliths externally visible under a high-power microscope as slight swellings.

The *leaves* (Fig. 1B, 2F) vary in size according to the robustness

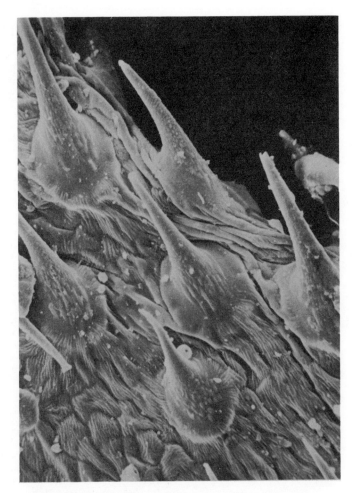

Fig. 4. Photograph (Stereoscan microscope) of hairs on upper surface of leaf of *Cannabis sativa*. Magnification x380. Photograph: Sims and Stearn.

of the plant. Each leaf has a slender stalk up to about 6 cm (2½ in.) long with a narrow groove along the upper side; in section the woody (vascular) tissue can be seen to form a continuous horseshoe- or U-shaped strand. The 3-11 (mostly 5-9) thin and soft-textured leaflets are mostly narrowly lanceolate (i.e. 6 or so times as long as broad and broadest below the middle), with a narrowly wedge-shaped

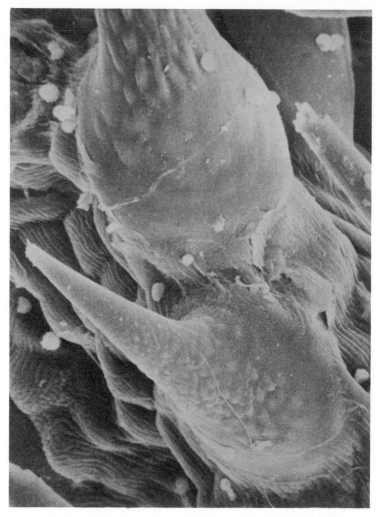

Fig. 5. Photograph (Stereoscan microscope) of hairs on lower
surface of leaf of *Cannabis sativa*. Magnification x850. Photograph:
Sims and Stearn.

base, a coarsely saw-toothed edge and a long drawn-out pointed tip;
the teeth, about 4-14 each side, are sharp and point towards the tip
of the leaflet; the veins run out obliquely from the midrib to the tips
of the teeth. The leaflets of a single leaf are uneven in size, with the

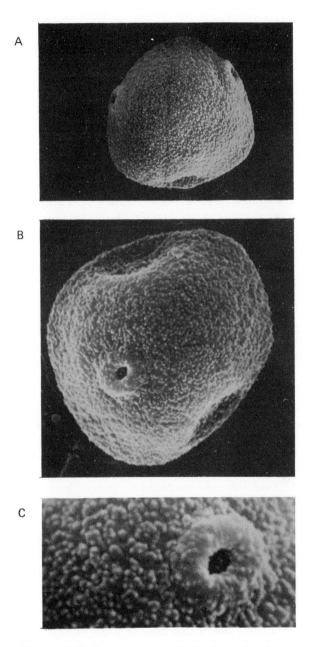

Fig. 6. Photograph (Stereoscan microscope) of pollen grains of *Cannabis sativa.* Magnification: A, ×3,000; B, ×5,000; and C, (pore) ×10,000. Photographs: Sims and Stearn.

largest up to 15 cm (6 in.) or so; they have very minute hairs on the
upper surface, more profuse and longer hairs 150-250 μ (about 1/125
in.) long on the lower surface. The hairs (trichomes) of the upper
surface (Fig. 3) have a globose base and a very short projecting point;
those of the lower surface (Figs. 4, 5) a less swollen base; they are all
unicellular, i.e. each formed of one cell.

The *flowers* (Figs. 1B, D, 2F, G) are produced in great abundance
on the upper part of the plant. A flower of *Cannabis* is unisexual,
i.e. it is either male (staminate) or female (pistillate). Usually an
individual plant bears only one kind of flower, i.e. it is wholly male
or wholly female, and the species is accordingly described as dioecious:
occasionally, however, male and female flowers occur on the same
individual and it is then described as monoecious. From a single
sowing, male and female individuals arise in about equal numbers but,
as male individuals are more conspicuous when in bloom than females,
male specimens are more frequently gathered by botanical collectors
than female ones and consequently are much better represented in
herbaria. Female plants are very leafy up to the top; male plants have
the leaves on the inflorescence fewer and much further apart. Male
plants die earlier than female plants and are often harvested earlier for
fibre or weeded out in order to get a bigger yield of resin from female
plants.

The *male inflorescence* (Fig. 1B) is loosely arranged, much-
branched and many-flowered, standing out from the leaves, with
individual flowering branches to 18 cm (7 in.) long; it is covered with
minute bristly hairs. Each flower (Fig. 1D) consists of 5 whitish or
greenish minutely hairy sepals (tepals or perigon segments) about
3.5 mm (1/8 in.) long and 5 pendulous stamens, with very slender
filaments and anthers (Fig. 1E) opening lengthwise from the tip
downwards to release the pollen which is carried by the wind to
female flowers. The pollen grains (Fig. 6) are almost circular in
outline, but slightly broader than long (oblate), about 25-30 μ
(*c.* 1/1000 in.) in diameter, smooth, with 2 to 4 circular germ-pores.

The *female inflorescences* (Fig. 2F) do not project beyond the
leaves; they are compact, short and few-flowered, with flowers borne
in pairs. The individual flower (Fig. 2G) has a small green organ, sometimes called a bract, sometimes a calyx (Fig. 2H, J), which completely enwraps the ovary and forms a basally swollen tubular sheath
about 1.8 mm-2.6 mm (about 1/12 in.) long, out of which project the

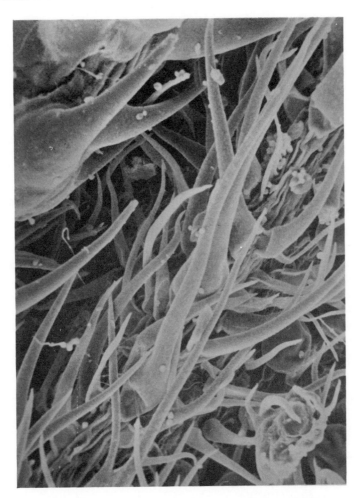

Fig. 7. Photograph (Stereoscan microscope) of hairs on bract of *Cannabis sativa* (♀). Magnification x340. Photograph: Sims and Stearn.

two stigmas. This sheath is covered with slender hairs (Fig. 7) and short-stalked or stalkless circular glands secreting drops of resin, which are produced most abundantly under hot conditions; in nature the function of these resin glands is presumably to protect the plant from animals. The female part (gynoecium) of the flower consists of a more or less globose ovary surmounted by two long slender pollen-catching stigmas (Fig. 2G). The ovary has one ovule; after pollination the stigmas quickly fall off but the sheath increases in size. The *fruit* (Fig. 2K) is technically an achene, i.e. it contains a single seed with a hard shell tightly covered by the thin wall of the ovary, the whole being regarded in practice as a "seed". This is ellipsoid, slightly compressed, smooth, about 2.5-5 cm (1/8-3/16 in.) long, 2-3.5 mm (1/10 in.) in diameter, greyish or brownish or variously patterned. The embryo (Fig. 2N) within the seed is strongly curved with the two seed-leaves (cotyledons) packed together along one side and the potential root (radicle) up the other, together with a small food-supply (endosperm); they contain much oil.

Cannabis and *Humulus* (hop) are the only two genera of the family *Cannabaceae*. They lack the milky juice characteristic of the family *Moraceae* (mulberry family) and have quite different fruits. The generic name *Cannabis* goes back to Roman times; the Latin word *cannabis* (Greek: κάνναβις) has accusative *cannabim*, genitive *cannabis*, ablative *cannabe*, and the now accepted family name *Cannabaceae* accordingly consists of the stem *Cannab-* plus the feminine plural adjectival ending *-aceae* (belonging to, have the nature of). The adjective *cannabinus* means "hemp-like". *Datisca cannabina* (family *Datiscaceae*) is a herbaceous perennial of hemp-like general appearance but with botanical characters quite different from those of *Cannabis*.

References

Lubbock, J., *A Contribution to our Knowledge of Seedlings* Vol. 2. London (1892).

Metcalfe, C. R. and Chalk, L., *Anatomy of the Dicotyledons* Vol. 2. Oxford: Clarendon Press (1950).

Miller, N. G., The Genera of *Cannabaceae* in the South-eastern United States. J. Arnold Arb 51: 185-203 (1970).

Purseglove, J. W., *Tropical Crops, Dicotyledons* Vol. 1. London: Longmans (1968).

Schreiber, A., Cannabis. In G. Hegi, *Illustrierte Flora von Mittel-Europa* 2te Aufl., 3. i: 290-295 Munich: Carl Hanser (1958).

Walter, H., Cannabis. In O. von Kirchner *et al., Lebensgeschichte der Blütenpflanzen Mitteleuropas* 2.i: 875-909. Stuttgart: Eugen Ulmer (1935).

Zindern Bakker, E. M. Van., *South African Pollen Grains and Spores* Part 1 Amsterdam and Cape Town: A. A. Balkema (1953).

2 Random Thoughts and Queries on the Botany of Cannabis

Richard Evans Schultes

"The hemp plant grows in a wild or spontaneous state over so wide an area, but at the same time is always so closely associated with places that are or may have been inhabited or used as trade routes, that it is difficult to say where it originated".

Watt (1889)

THE PLANT

It is a plant—this thing that we are about to discuss: a green plant, a very abundant and ubiquitous plant, an unusually valuable economic plant, possibly a dangerous plant, certainly in many ways a mysterious plant. Consequently, I am happy that this symposium, contrary to general procedure in such instances, will begin by considering the plant—some part of what we know about it, but, more important, some part of what we do not know botanically about it. For a thorough knowledge of *Cannabis sativa* as a plant must be basic to progress in studies of its derivatives and their significance to man and their effects on his life and social evolution. Its stature, its structure, its place, its life as a plant, these are all-important, and without a clear comprehension of them we flounder and are lost. So, let us now look at some aspects of this weedy organism as a plant. How much do we know? How little do we know?

The underlying theme of this symposium is, I believe, the consideration of what we really do not know or understand about *Cannabis* and its botany, chemistry and pharmacology. In fact what we do know and understand with certainty is much less than what still remains hidden in "a mist of uncertainty and conjecture". Oftentimes, indeed, we know far less about the botany of some of our important economic and agricultural plants than about some of the odd

11

and rare wild species of the Plant Kingdom. And of the major economic plants, *Cannabis* falls among those which, in many aspects of their botany, are least known—certainly an anomaly, in view of its antiquity, its diversity of uses and its success in spreading spontaneously over a large part of the earth's surface.

In a cursoiy panorama such as this talk must needs be, I cannot delve deeply into all of the poorly known or unknown aspects of the botany of *Cannabis*: first, for reasons of brevity; second, because I should consider primarily points bearing on the plant as the source of a narcotic; and third, because I must present the material in a form easily comprehended and pertinently meaningful to colleagues in chemistry, pharmacology and other fields of research often far removed from the plant itself. My principal aim is merely to stimulate thinking by presenting some of the unexplored aspects about *Cannabis* as a living, dynamic, complex chemical factory, concerning the life and evolution of which we should know more, whether we work with it in the laboratory as a dead, processed residue or in the field as an aggressive, plastic weed or cultigen. That so much is not known botanically may frustrate or discourage the chemist and pharmacologist, and justifiably so, but it is precisely such a danger that makes the interdisciplinary approach of this symposium so necessary and so fraught with potentialities.

EVALUATION

At the start, we might do well to emphasize several points basic to any evaluation of *Cannabis* and concerning which there is no doubt.

Cannabis sativa is a triple-purpose economic plant. It has served man long and well as the source of fibre from its stem; of an oil from its seeds; of a narcotic drug from its resin. This diversity of its utilitarian interest to man has been responsible, perhaps more than any other circumstance, for the extraordinary differentiation of the species into so many races or strains throughout its long asssociation with the human race.

The pericyclic bast fibre provides true hemp. Strong and durable, composed of 70% cellulose and reaching lengths of from 3 to 15 feet, it is chiefly a substitute for flax. The drying oil, a greenish yellow fluid of disagreeable flavour, finds employment mainly as a substitute for linseed oil in the paint and varnish industry, but it is of value also in

soap-making, while the oil-cake is used as cattle feed, and, in eastern
Europe especially, the seeds, containing sometimes up to 35% of oil,
are roasted and consumed by man. The narcotic properties reside in a
resin produced in glandular hairs on the leaves, stems and inflorescences.
A number of closely related chemical constituents in the resin are responsible for the euphoric, hallucinogenic and other biodynamic activity
of the several narcotic preparations of *Cannabis* which are eaten, drunk
or smoked.

There is now ethnobotanically no way of ascertaining definitively
which of these uses represents the earliest. Normally, however, the
uses of a plant proceed historically from the simpler to the more complex. If this holds for *Cannabis*—and I see no reason why it should
not—then we can assume that the plant was first valued in primitive
society as a source of fibre. This would obviously be the most easily
observed morphological characteristic of the plant, a characteristic
which, when the stems rotted or were naturally retted, would have
been difficult or impossible for man in an inquisitive stage of cultural
development to have overlooked. We do know, from archaeological
evidence, that in Europe and the near East, at least, the employment
of *Cannabis* as a fibre source was perhaps the most ancient of the three
uses. Next to have been discovered, perhaps, might have been the
curiously narcotic effects of the resin when it was ingested—for we
know that man in primitive societies experiments orally with almost
any if not all plant tissues. We might logically argue that, at least in
some regions, the narcotic use could have preceded all others, since
magic is the essence of man's spiritual development, especially in
primitive societies. The unearthly effects of the drug must early have
assumed a magico-religious importance. The last and probably much
more recent discovery could have been the value of the oil expressed
from the seeds.

One supporting reason for this presumed sequence might be the
geographical extent of these several uses. The use of *Cannabis* to
produce fibre is more widespread than its employment as a narcotic
or medicine which, in turn, is diffused over a larger area than the
utilization of the seed as a source of oil.

HISTORY

Whichever may have been its earliest economic significance, *Cannabis* does represent one of man's oldest useful cultivated plants. In fact, I believe that it may represent actually one of our oldest non-food plants. Knowledge of its use by man goes back at least 6,000 years, and obviously man valued it long before our earliest records were made or our oldest archaeological remains were preserved. Archaeological specimens have been found in an Egyptian site of 3,000 to 4,000 years of age. Hempen fabrics have been excavated in sites near Ankara, Turkey, dated in the late 8th Century B.C. The Scythians, who burned *Cannabis* seed to produce an intoxicating smoke, grew hemp in the Volga region some 3,000 years ago. The plant was cultivated in Palestine and Mesopotamia at the time of Christ, but the earliest Roman mention of it was made about 100 B.C. Chinese tradition puts its date back some 4,800 years when Emperor Shen-Nung is credited with teaching his people to cultivate the plant for fibre. Although its value as a fibre plant dates back much earlier, the Indian medical writings, especially the Susrita, compiled before 1,000 B.C., report the therapeutic utilization of *Cannabis* resin, and as the nature of some of the vernacular names in India indicates, its narcotic properties were appreciated in the earliest Hindu writings.

Coarse hempen cloth, sometimes estimated to be 6,000 years of age, has turned up in some of the oldest sites of human habitation in Europe. Hempen textiles have been found in Romano-Gallic sites near Cologne, Germany, of the 3rd Century A.D. Seeds and leaves of *Cannabis,* indicating possibly its employment as a food, have been identified from a receptacle excavated near Berlin, Germany, and dated, albeit with some doubt, at about 500 B.C. Archaeological and historical evidence for early England is sparse, but specimens of hempen rope have been recovered from a Roman fort dated 140-180 A.D. In fact, there is very little evidence that *Cannabis* was cultivated, at least as a major plant, in western Europe before the Christian era, but from about 500 A.D. onward, the indications that it was, at least locally, an important crop plant in westernmost Europe are more abundant and trustworthy.

Palynological evidence, as shown by Godwin (1967), has been very helpful in tracing the path of *Cannabis* in western Europe and England and gives hope for similar studies elsewhere. A pollen diagram from an East Anglian lake, for example, indicated that from early Anglo-Saxon times there is a continuous curve for pollen of *Cannabis sativa* cultivated in ever-increasing amounts into late Saxon and Norman times.

Cannabis was introduced first to North America, north of Mexico, apparently by the Pilgrims of New England about 1632.

ORIGINS

There appears to be general agreement that *Cannabis sativa* is an Old World plant, unknown in the Western Hemisphere before the 16th Century. No botanist has ever doubted this opinion, which has been held from the time of Linnaeus' formal naming of the species to Alphonse de Candolle's recognition of the Old and New World assemblages of cultivated plants as distinct and to the modern concepts of Vavilov, Schwanitz, Zhukovskii and other specialists on plant domestication.

There appears, furthermore, to be general agreement that *Cannabis* is Asiatic, and little doubt that it arrived comparatively late in Europe. Writing about 450 B.C., Herodotus stated that hemp "grows in Scythia; it is very like flax, only that it is a much taller and coarser plant. Some grows wild about the country; some is produced by cultivation . . . The Scythians take some of this hemp seed, and, creeping under felt coverings, throw it upon the red-hot stones; immediately it smokes and gives out such a vapour as no Grecian bath can excel". Most authorities feel that hemp was introduced into western Europe about 1500 B.C. by the Scythian invaders from Asia, that it did not come into Europe through the Mediterranean countries of the classical period, where it remained comparatively unknown until just prior to the beginning of the Christian Era. The plant was obviously spread westward in Europe by Teutonic peoples, as indicated in part by linguistic evidence. Most probably it was reintroduced to Europe many times and from sundry sources, if we may judge from the variety of races of the plant cultivated and spontaneous in different regions of Europe. It seems difficult to explain all the many races and their distribution on climatic or environmental selection alone. Boyce wonders, for example, if there might not have been an indigenous variety or race of hemp in Celtic Europe that crossed with one that was introduced originally from the Himalayan region. This is a unique, even though rather unorthodox idea, and one well worth considering, in view of the near-impossibility of explaining the complexity of modern European hemp on the basis of other factors alone.

Let us return, in greater detail, to the problem of where *Cannabis* originated, because if our experience in other economic crop plants be a reliable guide, this aspect is basically and even perhaps exclusively important in understanding the plant in its present ubiquitous occurrence and complex diversity.

It is not always easy to distinguish between wild, spontaneous, semi-cultivated, and cultivated plants. As Vavilov points out, specialists who have written on the occurrence of *Cannabis* in central Asia have had to employ such terms as *quasi-spontanea, subspontanea, spontanea videtur, erratica* when they were not certain, while others aggressively described that plant as *spontaneous, wild, running wild, almost wild,* or *escaped.* As a result, the literature might give the impression that hemp was "wild" over a greater area than really is true. I believe that we should use the term "wild" for a plant only when it grows wholly without man's care in what is thought to be its native area and that, in other regions, the terms *spontaneous* or *adventitious* might more appropriately be employed. But, as we search the literature of *Cannabis*, we must guard against the report of its growing "wild", because of the generally uncritical use of this term.

There is no agreement—except within extraordinarily large areas of Asia—as to where *Cannabis* really originated. Some authors assert that it is indigenous to the temperate parts of Asia near the Caspian Sea, southern Siberia, and the Kirghiz Desert, possibly including also parts of Persia. Other authorities have suggested northern India and the Himalayas. Alphonse de Candolle, the first serious student of the origin of cultivated plants, specifies that "the species has been found wild, beyond a doubt, to the south of the Caspian Sea, near the Irtysch, in the desert of Kirghiz, beyond Lake Baikal in Dahuria . . . Authors mention it throughout southern and central Russia and to the south of the Caucasus, but its wild nature is here less certain . . . The antiquity of the cultivation of hemp in China leads me to believe", he continues, "that its area extends further to the east, although this has not yet been proved by botanists."

Vavilov's meticulous work—a combination of critical sifting of the literature and extensive field observations—has accepted this general area. Zhukovskii, however, favours an area of origin in the Himalayas.

In connexion with the consideration of the native area of *Cannabis*, these three specialists handled the classification of the species very differently. De Candolle did not discuss variants of *Cannabis sativa* in his arguments. Vavilov insisted on recognizing the weedy hemp that has "run wild" as a true wild plant with characters sufficiently clear to single it out confidently as a variety—*Cannabis sativa* var. *spontanea*—distinct from the cultivated type. Zhukovskii goes further in this direction, considering the weedy hemp occurring in a wild or spontaneous state in the steppes and cultivated fields of the upper and lower Volga region, western Siberia and central Asia and now spreading, he says, into more northern parts of European Russia, as a distinct species, *Cannabis ruderalis*. The cultivated hemp, which, he maintains, grows wild and as an escape in the Trans-Volga region, on the islands of the Volga Delta, in the mountains of Altai and Caucasus, and especially in Azerbaijan, as well as in the Himalayas, Hindu-Kush and Mongolia, he refers to as *Cannabis sativa*. He points out, however, that Nikiforov recognized taxonomically two races of the escaped, weedy form of this species: one large-fruited, the other small-fruited, with monoecious strains in both. The third species accepted by Zhukovskii, *Cannabis indica*, represents the plant cultivated for narcotic products in India, Iran, Turkey, Syria and North Africa and occurring "wild" in Pakistan and Kafiristan.

Obviously, neither Vavilov nor Zhukovskii envisage genetically stable "*varietates*" in these concepts, since both indicate that the main argument in their decisions concerning the origin of cultivated hemp is that this plant, even to-day, especially in central Asia, can be found in a truly wild state. Zhukovskii further supports his decisions with the belief that the species *Cannabis ruderalis* and *C. indica* cannot be ancestral types of the cultivated *C. sativa*. Mansfeld recognizes still different categories: *Cannabis indica* in India (especially northwestern India), Iran and eastern Afghanistan; and *C. sativa* with two sub-species: wild or cultivated subspecies, *spontanea* (or *C. ruderalis*) of Altai, Tienshan, Transcaucasia, Afghanistan, the Balkans and middle Europe; and *culta*, indigenous to Asia (northern Himalayas and Hindu-Kush to China), Europe, North Africa, North and South America, Australia.

It would seem that historical and ethnobotanical evidence must have greater weight perhaps—at least at the present state of our understanding—than the study of collections of wild, cultivated or spontaneous specimens. We must come to this conclusion in view of the diverse results that careful consideration of field data have led to in their evaluation by such scholars as Vavilov and Zhukovskii.

I cannot here refrain from emphasizing my conviction that much more thorough and critical search for an unquestionably wild and ancestral form of *Cannabis* must be attempted before we can truly

understand the modern cultigen. Vavilov's monumental work is now
fully a third of a century behind us. Techniques for comprehension
of the factors involved in plant domestication have greatly improved
during the past few decades. Furthermore, methods of ecology are
now far more sophisticated. Is it visionary to suggest that we re-examine
the populations of *Cannabis* where we believe ancestral forms still thrive?

We are left without any very definite region for the origin of *Cannabis
sativa* as a domesticate. This—like other critical aspects of the total
study of the hemp plant—is intricately involved with a clearer study
of its classification, its genetics and cytology and its ecology. I also
strongly believe that a clear chemotaxonomic understanding of this
important and possibly sinister economic plant must be sought. This
may, in turn, aid in unravelling some of these mysteries, when we look
at *Cannabis sativa* through less compartmentalized and monodisciplinary
sights and when we go back to an analytical study of ancestral types.

DOMESTICATION

Wherever *Cannabis* may have been native, the problem of how it was
domesticated still remains for us to consider. An understanding of
this process bears directly on certain contemporary experimental
enquiries into the behaviour of *Cannabis*.

How did early man begin domestication of plants? It is reasonable
to suppose that the earliest steps in the case of both plants and animals were largely accidental. Early man did not sit down and muse:
"Now I have reached a stage in culture when it behooves me to invent
agriculture". He was probably led—perhaps almost forced—to the
domestication of plants, especially his food plants, and by circumstances largely fortuitous. There must have been a gradual transition
from the gathering of wild plants to the growing of cultivated ones.

We do have evidence from primitive yet still living cultures that
this transition takes place. One of the best examples is in *Cannabis*.
It is found in many parts of the world both cultivated and spontaneous.
The spontaneous hemp is presumably escaping from the cultivated
types. The reverse trend can likewise take place—cultivated types are
being domesticated from wild or spontaneous hemps. This two-way
shift is, of course, recognized as taking place in other economic plants,
notably in rice in India.

Wild and spontaneous *Cannabis* is not identical with cultivated hemp: its seeds are smaller; most plants are deciduous, scattering their seed; many of the seeds have delayed germination.

Hemp does best on a fertile, well drained soil. It is a heavy feeder and a soil-depleting crop. The high fertility requirements of *Cannabis* are so notorious that in Italy where fine hemp fibre is grown there is a proverb that "it will *grow* anywhere, but without manure will be fit for no use, though planted in heaven itself". Darlington calls hemp a "dung hill plant"; Edgar Anderson, a typical "camp follower".

Whatever we call it, *Cannabis* not only prefers but almost demands rich soils and, as a consequence, encroaches naturally on man's dwelling space where rubbish, garbage and excrement accumulate. Man will then eventually recognize the value of the fibres and oil of the plant growing in his very dooryard, especially in times of food shortage, and soon he will himself be sowing and caring for it. Disturbances of natural habitats have been greatly accelerated since man began to live on the earth; and he has constantly created new ecological niches for plants either native to the area or brought with him in his restless rovings from unfamiliar and foreign environments. "As he unconsciously bred the quick-growing weeds capable of utilizing soils high in nitrogen, he also unconsciously carried them about from place to place and gave them previously unparalleled opportunities to . . . build up into super-weeds". Domesticated hemp definitely started in this way. Under cultivation, the large-seeded, non-deciduous forms—the seed of which all germinates simultaneously—forms arising from mutation—are at a distinct advantage. These soon replace the small-seeded forms with delayed or variable germination. It is really not even necessary for man to select for this character himself. These steps in domestication of hemp have been observed and reported by Vavilov in Altai in central Asia. Many of the other characteristics brought to the fore in cultivated forms—absence of a large perianth and thin seed coat—are recessive characters.

The domestication of *Cannabis* came about probably in several localities more or less simultaneously, as indicated by the great diversity of geographical and morphological types amongst cultivated forms. The germ plasm represented by these numerous types must have been very ample to have permitted, in subsequent times, the extraordinary morphological plasticity that we now see in *Cannabis* and its almost unique geographical and climatic adaptability over a great part of the world.

Palynology has been helpful in tracing the path of *Cannabis* as a domesticate and has shown that it was cultivated for fibre and oil in western Asia some 900 years B.C.

TAXONOMY

The life of *Cannabis* in modern botanical nomenclature and taxonomy began when Linnaeus set up the genus in 1735. It was based, however, on pre-Linnean concepts, and the name *Cannabis* itself was taken from ancient vernacular usage going back even to Sanskrit roots.

It would be extremely interesting to review the ancient literature concerning the hemp plant. Until the 17th Century, botany and medicine in European literature were, for all practical purposes, one. Consequently, all of the ancient literature would be medico-botanical. However, we cannot here take time for an excursion into this earlier phase of *Cannabis* literature but must be content with a passing mention of Dioscorides' discussion of the plant, in the 1st Century A.D. as, translated by Goodyer: "Cannabis is a plant of much use in this life for ye twistings of very strong ropes, it bears leaves like to the Ash, of a bad scent, long stalks, empty, a round seed, which being eaten of much doth quench geniture, but being juiced when it is green is good for the pains of the ears". This description, like those of most if not all of the early medico-botanical writers, stresses the useful qualities of the plant and lacks almost wholly the morphological details upon which modern botany has built its systems of classification. The conspicuous absence of any references to the intoxicating qualities of the plant do not fail to engage the reader's attention, however, and it is generally believed that at this early period knowledge of the narcotic use of *Cannabis* had not reached the Mediterranean area.

Even more significant is the lack of mention of any narcotic properties in Rabelais's remarkably detailed account in 1546 of the celebrated 'Pantagruelion' herb (Book 3, chapters 49-51), i.e. hemp, wherein he refers to the seeds beloved by finches and also eaten by Greeks and its fibres hated by robbers which made them end their lives high and quickly. Had even a hint of its hallucinogenic powers reached that inquisitive and exuberant scholar, he would certainly have expounded such exciting matters at length.

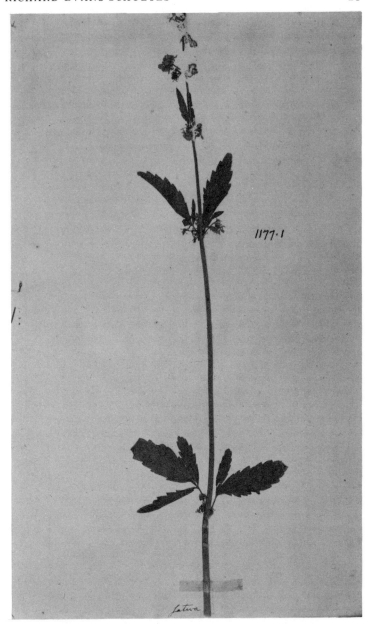

Fig. 1. Specimen No. 1177.1 of *Cannabis sativa* L. in the Linnean
Herbarium. Courtesy: Linnean Society of London.

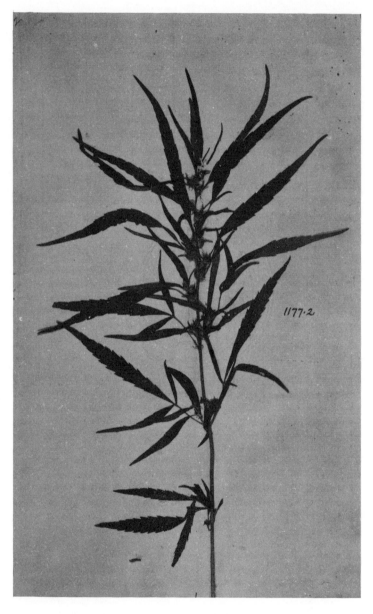

Fig. 2. Specimen No. 1177.2 of *Cannabis sativa* L. in the Linnean Herbarium. Courtesy: Linnean Society of London.

The name *Cannabis sativa* was used by Caspar Bauhin in 1623 but its first publication as a deliberate binomial dates from Linnaeus's *Species Plantarum* of 1753, which is the internationally accepted starting point for modern botanical nomenclature. Linnaeus listed under this binomial several pre-Linnaean synonyms: his own *Cannabis foliis digitatis* used in his *Hortus Cliffortianus* (1738), *C. sativa* and *C. erratica* of Caspar Bauhin (1623), *C. mas* and *C. femina* of D'Aléchamps (1587).

The Linnean Society of London preserves in Linnaeus' herbarium two specimens of *Cannabis sativa*. One specimen, No. 1177.1 (Fig. 1), is labelled *"sativa"* in Linnaeus' handwriting and represents a staminate plant, with much more abbreviated leaves than is usual in the genus. No. 1177.2 (Fig. 2), without a specific epithet written on the sheet, represents a pistillate plant with the lanceolate leaves that are normal for the species. There are, of course, no locality data on these two specimens, although in *Species Plantarum*, Linnaeus offers the information that the species has a "habitat in India". In his annotated copy of *Species Plantarum*, which is preserved at the Linnean Society, Linnaeus had written, in his own hand, as a note for a further edition, the word "Persia" as an additional habitat.

Botanists now generally agree that *Cannabis* is a monotypic genus, a genus with one species: *C. sativa*; that there cannot be recognized any true botanical varieties within this species; and that this one species has diversified into a great number of ecotypes and cultivated races. Modern taxonomists, thus, are in agreement with Linnaeus' treatment of the genus.

Nevertheless, a number of binomials have been legitimately published for distinct concepts once thought to deserve nomenclatorial recognition. These are *Cannabis chinensis* Delile; *C. erratica* Siev.; *C. foetens* Gilib.; *C. indica* Lam.; *C. Lupulus* Scop.; *C. macrosperma* Stokes; *C. americana* Pharm. ex Wehmer; *C. generalis* E. H. L. Krause; *C. gigantea* Crevost; *C. ruderalis* Janischevskii; and a hybrid, *C. X interstitia* Sojak.

As early as 1869, de Candolle recognized several varieties of *Cannabis sativa*, offering very detailed descriptions of each one: α *Kif;* β *vulgaris;* γ *Pedemontana;* δ *Chinensis.*

Although none of these is accepted by most modern taxonomists, confusion of nomenclature still reigns in the non-technical literature.

In agricultural, horticultural, chemical and pharmacological publi-

cations, it is not uncommon to find in use Latin binomials that have
no validity, since they were never validly published. The binomial
Cannabis indica is, however, frequently employed as though it represented a species-concept distinct from *C. sativa* and most often to
indicate a race native to India and usually high in concentration of
intoxicating principles. Even more frequently, pharmacological
writings use the name *Cannabis sativa* var. *indica* in the belief that
there exists a definitive "*varietas*" of Indian origin that may be dis-
tinquished taxonomically by having a higher content of the narcotic
constituents: a physiological race or chemovar which, it is often
asserted, cannot long be maintained in an inappropriate climate and
environment. Some have gone even beyond this to distinguish nomen-
clatorially other varieties. There is still so much confusion that some
pharmacological reports have even used the epithets "*Cannabis indica*"
and "*C. sativa* var. *indica*" as though the two were distinct concepts!

Morphological or taxonomic botanists cannot accept true varieties
within *Cannabis sativa*, simply because they cannot define them. On
the basis of cytological studies, Postma concluded that there was only
one species which might be split into many kinds of "subspecies", but
that perhaps it might be better to speak of two types of *Cannabis
sativa*: the northern, to which the Russian hemps might be relegated;
and the southern, to which belong the Indian hemps. Agricultural and
horticultural specialists are prone to recognize different species and
varieties, but admit that they are not stable. We are here speaking
about two very distinct concepts: the true "*varietas*", which is genetically distinct; and the non-genetical response to environmental and
other factors, concepts which are better called "races", "ecotypes",
"cultivars", "chemovars" or other appropriate terms.

One of the most succinct summaries—and this from an agriculturist,
not from a taxonomist—is that of the American fibre specialist, Dewey.
"Hemp, cultivated for three different products", he wrote, "has developed into three rather distinct types of groups of forms. The extreme .
forms of each group have been described as different species, but the
presence of intergrading forms and the fact that the types do not
remain distinct . . . under new conditions make it impossible to regard
them as valid species. There are few recognized varieties in either
group. Less than 20 varieties of fibre-producing hemp are known,
although hemp has been cultivated for more than 40 centuries, or
much longer than either cotton or corn, both of which now have
hundreds of named varieties".

One cause of the chaos in taxonomic and nomenclatorial recognition of polymorphism in *Cannabis sativa* has been misunderstanding of species delimitation in cultivated plants. No botanist can draw a sharp line between a cultivated and a wild or spontaneous plant. It is probable that most of the changes that occur with cultivated plants occur likewise in the wild representatives. True species do occur amongst cultigens; but, with cultivated forms, the differences, in contrast to those recognized in wild or spontaneous populations, are usually minor and often not of a genetic or hereditary nature. These minor variations often have agricultural, commercial or other practical significance and, consequently, may be considered of greater importance than more basic differences in wild populations. It is often most convenient to distinguish a cultigen by glorifying it with a binomial, with the result that there have been, as indicated previously, many Latin binomials applied to cultigens.

The recognition of races, ecotypes and other kinds of convivia with Latin designations in the rank of species for convenience confuses classification, since the minor concepts—e.g. *Cannabis indica*—are not the equivalent of a Linnean species. Vavilov pointed out that the study of cultivated plants ". . . sometimes made it necessary to postulate late large Linnaean species. We are coming to the concept of a Linnaean species as a definite, discrete, dynamic system differentiated into geographical and ecological types and comprising sometimes an enormous number of varieties". Even these "geographical" and "ecological types" cannot be treated as true botanical varieties.

VARIATIONS

It is now quite generally accepted that *Cannabis* tends to resemble or differ from a parental or ancestral strain according to environmental conditions under which it is grown. Is this really invariably true, however, or are a few striking examples being overemphasized? Have controlled experiments on a large scale ever been done to back up this belief? And what are the kinds of difference—morphological, physiological, chemical, etc.—that are connected with phytobiotic factors? What are the principal environmental factors that do influence this polymorphism: climatic factors, such as sunlight, length of day, wind, variation in humidity; lithospheric and hydrospheric influences like water content, nutritive content, temperature and other characteristics of the soil; vegetational factors, such as humus formation; and pyric factors of both the anthropeic and non-anthropeic or natural environment?

The plasticity of *Cannabis* has long been recognized but has never been truly understood. Charles Darwin was impressed by this aggressive weed. Plants long cultivated "can", he wrote, "generally endure with undiminished fertility various and great changes", and hemp may be "so much affected that the proportions and the nature of their chemical ingredients are modified". The *Report of the Indian Hemp Drugs Commission* attempted in 1894 to set forth definitive thoughts on this aspect of the plant after an exhaustive survey by questionnaire. It stated that in India the only differences recognized by the people (and botanists should heed folk classifications more frequently) are between the *wild* and *cultivated* plant, the male and female plants and certain colour differences; and that, while the inherent potentiality of the seed to develop a plant closely resembling the parents must be admitted, there is no evidence of racial speciality or differentiation of definitive forms. In India, the Commission found, the plant cultivated for fibre yields the narcotic, and evidence was strong that the wild plant also yields the intoxicating resin. *Cannabis* grown for production of the narcotic *ganja* or *bhang* yielded fibre as well, even though, in India, fibre production was a very limited activity. Chopra and Chopra write that "even the plant growing under different climatic conditions in the vast Indo-Pakistan sub-continent shows remarkable variations in appearance; those variations at first may give the impression of separate species".

The plasticity of *Cannabis* was shown experimentally by Christison and Hope as early as 1847, by J. Bouquet in 1912 and, more recently, by others: plants grown in England and France from seed imported from India were, after several generations, morphologically indistinguishable from the races long acclimatized to European conditions. Further experiments indicated that conversely the same holds true of European material planted out for several generations in dry, warm areas such as Egypt and Tunisia. Another interesting indication of this susceptibility to environment is the experience in Egypt when hemp seed procured from Europe and planted to supply cordage for an incipient navy soon changed, making it imperative to import new seed periodically, since the quality of the fibre steadily degenerated, while the plants began to produce more and more intoxicating resin.

Although the pharmaceutical literature long persisted—and still often does so—in recognizing the Indian *Cannabis* as distinct, botanists such as Watt early pointed out that although " the European form of the plant was supposed to be distinct from the Asiatic, the chief value of the latter consisting in its narcotic properties . . . this distinction has now disappeared from the literature of the subject, since it could not be supported by botanical characters. The reduction became the more necessary when it was fully understood that, according to climate and soil, the Indian plant varied in as marked a degree as it differed from the European". Watt further pointed out that *Cannabis sativa*, in high mountainous areas of India, yields a superb fibre; that, in Kashmir, it was valued for the resin exuding from the stem and leaves just before maturation of the flowers; that, in the plains, instead of secreting resin from splits in the bark, the plant produces it in the young pistillate flowers and twigs; that, in other parts of India, the narcotic principle is not developed until the fertilized ovaries are nearly mature. "We have here", Watt says, " . . . one of the most notable illustrations of the effect of climate in changing the chemical processes . . . of a plant".

For a long while, the *United States Pharmacopoeia* insisted that medically active hemp coud be supplied officially only by the Indian plant or *"Cannabis indica"*. The 8th edition of the *Pharmacopoeia*, for example, specified that *"Cannabis indica* shall consist of the dried prepared tops of the pistillate plant of *Cannabis sativa* grown in the East Indies . . .". So far afield did the pharmaceutical literature stray that the *National Standard Dispensatory* reported that "the rich soil and cool climate suitable for the production of hemp fibre will not develop the medicinal properties . . .".

Following a spirited argument in the literature, Hamilton and others showed conclusively that American-grown hemp did contain the active constituents; that, if equal care were exercised in selecting the proper part of the drug for extraction, no material difference in activity would be found between Indian and American hemp; and that, since *Cannabis* grown in various localities in the United States and Mexico was fully as active as the best imported Indian material, there was no valid reason why American hemp could not replace the imported Asiatic product. Furthermore, the work of Sabalitschka indicated that high resin content perhaps may not wholly be due to climate, since seeds of common European hemp taken to India failed there to produce a higher resin content.

While these and other specialists can cite statistical studies to the contrary, there is ample evidence, equally reliable, that *Cannabis sativa* does indeed change drastically, though impermanently, in response to environmental factors. Adams, for example, asserted that "the amount of resin depends almost entirely on the climate, the largest . . . in hot dry climates such as Chinese Turkestan and the smallest in temperate climates where there is plenty of moisture". I could cite any number of additional specialists who accept this contention, and I tend to believe it to be true, with certain limitations, although large-scale controlled plantings alone can experimentally answer these questions with finality; and apparently such experiments have never been carried out. They may never be attempted. It is to be hoped, however, that they will be— not only because of the immediate understanding of a plant that, although important to man, may become a danger to his health and well-being, but because of the insights that such a study will provide for a fuller understanding of some of our other basic economic plants. It is here that the joint efforts, fully integrated, of botanists, ecologists, agronomists, horticulturists, chemotaxonomists, phytochemists and pharmacologists are sorely needed.

It is obvious that what has interested certain investigators most avidly is the possible creation of chemovars with high concentration of the intoxicating principles. What about gross morphology? There seems, from the reliable literature, to be every probability that environmental conditions can influence rapidly and significantly the morphology of the plant. Adams, for example, is very explicit about this point when he says that "the morphological characters . . . are modified very easily—one variety to another—merely by a change in climatic conditions". It is very definitely known, for example, that the tallest forms of fibre-yielding *Cannabis sativa* are produced in China and Japan, where the plants have slender, sparesely branched internodes 8 to 10 inches long; that the European types have shorter, more rigid stems and require two weeks less time to mature than the Asiatic forms. There seems, on the surface, to be little doubt that this is true— but again: what *are* the changes induced and what *factors* are active in bringing about these modifications? Camp grew, under controlled conditions, a number of so-called varieties, the original seed of which came from different parts of the world. Sown in adjacent plots over several years in garden and greenhouse, they showed difference in size, time of flowering, seed productivity, fibre quality and drug content; but, except for one known mutant, he found no difference sufficiently stable and important to separate them into distinct groups. One proof of the truly monotypic nature of *Cannabis* is this basic similarity in forms, despite its cultivation and differential selection by various and widespread racial groups since antiquity.

One aspect of the polymorphism resulting from the plasticity of *Cannabis* and which, I believe, is not sufficiently stressed in the agricultural and botanical literature has to do with its manipulation by man for so long a time. *Cannabis* is such an ancient economic plant, has been subjected over so many millenia by man to subconscious and conscious selection, that a bewildering array of cultivars has appeared. Obviously many of the cultivars that have appeared have disappeared. When man was interested primarily in production of a strong and long fibre, selection tended to proceed along lines that would produce cultivars with superior fibres; and the same has been true in parts of the world where a major interest was directed towards greater intoxicating properties. It is often the case that, when a plant is intensively selected for one characteristic, other characteristics suffer or even disappear. In *Cannnabis sativa*, races of unusually high yield of seed oil or superior fibre have been developed which are either inferior in narcotic principles or wholly devoid of them—yet these races are reported as growing in the same region, sometimes even in adjacent fields! On the contrary, highly narcotic races are reported in which the quality of fibre is decidedly inferior, so much so that these strains are commercially worthless—yet they may, too, grow in the same region. Do we really know—are we really certain—that the deductions from uncontrolled commercial plantings that have led to these propositions are reliable and definitive? Have scientists made these pronouncements—or are they promulgated by production managers and government statistics agents? Or have the results of what experimental data we do have been interpreted under the shadow of prejudice from what we know in the case of other cultivated plants? Is it wise to assume that *Cannabis* will follow the norms of other cultivated plants in its much more complicated, geographically more extensive and economically more diverse nature? These are basic questions that we must consider, if we are to learn more about the plant and its idiosyncrasies. Much of a basic nature certainly remains for scientists to authenticate along these lines, yet we must always bear in mind that in *Cannabis sativa* it will be hard—especially in cultivated and even escaped or spontaneous populations—to avoid the results of the complicating finger of man.

There is one point, however, on which we can here be certain: the inadvisability of using technical Latin nomenclature to designate the minor variants of *Cannabis sativa*. It is, of course, accepted practice in horticulture and agriculture to designate definite cultivars with vernacular names. Many of the cultivars of *Cannabis sativa* have been so designated. Man has selected hundreds of strains, races or other types of cultivars during the millenia that he has had to manipulate this economic plant, and in modern times he has engaged in conscious and purposeful selection. Until recently, hemp has been essentially a cultivated wild plant, but through appropriate modern methods and selection, the fibre content has been increased 100% in some strains, up to 200% in others. The greatest emphasis, naturally, has been given to the variants of hemp as a fibre plant, but selection has had effects also in strains for narcotic constituents and for oil content.

A number of named variants of hemp are recognised, especially in the fibre industry. Although the statement that there are 20 or fewer "varieties" of *Cannabis* cultivated for fibre is often quoted, there are in reality many more. The fibre hemp grown in the United States in colonial times was of European origin, but the type basic to modern American fibre production—commonly known as "Kentucky"—was originally from China. Selection for improved fibre quality and production has been carried on in a number of countries. In the United States, for example, it has resulted in at least one widely grown cultivar called "Kymington". In Europe, five or six varieties are considered outstanding. A recent chemical and biological evaluation of the resin of hemp grown for seed in Russia enumerates 19 named "varieties". More attention must, however, be given to the classification of these agronomic variants. The need for an intensive study of this kind on highly intoxicating races in India is most to be desired.

CLASSIFICATION

In the classification of such an ancient, economically diversified and geographically extended plant, one might be justified in expecting some taxonomic accord as to its position in the dicotyledons. One may well be dismayed that we still have not reached universal agreement about the family position of *Cannabis*.

Cannabis is closely allied to *Humulus*, the genus of the hop plant.

Botanists group them together, usually with *Cannabis* as a monotypic genus and *Humulus* with three species, although some authorities believe that all three of the species of *Humulus* are referable to *H. lupulus*.

Early taxonomists tended to place *Cannabis* and *Humulus* in the *Urticaceae* or Nettle Family, although it was not uncommon, early in the 19th Century, to find the genus collocated in the *Moraceae* or Fig Family. Both families belong, of course, to the Order *Urticales* and are, to be sure, closely related. A number of earlier botanists felt constrained to create for *Cannabis* and *Humulus* a distinct family: *Cannabaceae* or Hempwort Family, still accommodated in the *Urticales* and patently allied to both the *Urticaceae* and the *Moraceae*. The family name is sometimes written *Cannabiaceae*, *Cannabidaceae* or, most often, *Cannabinaceae*. When *Cannabis* and *Humulus* were included within the *Urticaceae* or the *Moraceae*, however, a separate subfamily or other sectional distinction (e.g. *Cannaboideae*) was usually made. Whatever we call these two genera—separate family or section of *Urticaceae* or *Moraceae*—there is evidence that they are evolutionarily relatively highly advanced.

If I were to generalize, I would say that the earliest trend in taxonomic works was to include *Cannabis* in the *Urticaceae*; that in the last half of the last century and the early part of this century, most authorities favoured the *Moraceae*; that the modern tendency appears to maintain the family *Cannabaceae* as separate from these. Recent studies in morphology and chemistry likewise support the separation of *Cannabis* into a distinct family. In modern agricultural and horticultural writings, *Cannabis* is usually assigned to the *Moraceae*.

Even though in writing about *Cannabis* as a narcotic I have myself usually preferred to assign it to the *Moraceae*, I must agree that a critical evaluation of the taxonomic characters convinces me that there is ample evidence on which to accept the *Cannabaceae* as a discrete family concept that represents—in *Cannabis* and *Humulus*—a distinct trend in urticalean evolution and that there is both a morphological and chemical basis for this point of view.

The *Cannabaceae* appear to be more closely allied to the *Urticaceae* than to the *Moraceae*, although in many respects this small family is intermediate between the other two larger families. Hegnauer intimates, from chemical evidence, a closer alliance with *Moraceae*.

From the *Urticaceae,* it differs in its erect (instead of inflexed or

coiled) anther filament in bud; in its hanging (instead of erect) ovule;
in the aromatic quality of the plants; and in the lack of stinging hairs,
while urticaceous plants often possess urticant pilosity. These represent
major and basically significant differences.

The *Cannabaceae* differ from the *Moraceae* most conspicuously in
the form of flowers and fruit; in the latter, the flowers are numerous
on or inside a large receptacle and the achenes are enclosed in a fleshy
calyx or are aggregated into a spherical mass or else borne inside a
large fleshy or leathery receptacle that forms usually a hollow fruit
known as a cynconium or fig; in the former, the flowers are not borne
on the inside of a receptacle, and the sepals are not fleshy nor do they
envelop the achene in fruit. These, too, are meaningful differences.
The *Moraceae* are nearly all trees and shrubs with conspicuous milky
latex, whereas the *Cannabaceae* are herbs or vines, not woody, and are
devoid of a milky latex, although *Cannabis* does have unbranched,
unicellular latex vessels.

There is still much to resolve regarding the taxonomic position
and relationships of *Cannabis*, but only a fundamental integration of
morphology, anatomy, cytology and chemistry with what is now
known taxonomically can take us nearer to a meaningful understanding
of the true phylogenetic position of this anomalous plant.

There are many problems demanding study in a variety of aspects
of the botany of *Cannabis*. I have been derelict in not delving into
many of them, but they are too numerous and complex to discuss
lightly. Ecology—especially as it concerns the spread of spontaneous
hemp and its successful survival as a weed—will certainly be most
illuminating once a basic program is started. Just what is the secret of
the aggressiveness of *Cannabis*? How much of the success that this
plant has had in spreading can be attributed to chemical or other
characteristics of the soil? What effect do fungal, insect or other
diseases have on its spread? Why does it do better under drier conditions? Although preliminary cytological studies have been carried
out, showing that this 20-chromosome species is an allopolyploid,
more intensive and extensive investigations may throw much light on
the taxonomic position and biology of *Cannabis sativa*. We have really
considered little or nothing of the tremendous variation in chemical
constituents—the intoxicating principles and sundry others—in relation
to the total life of the plant. What, if anything, does the botany of
Cannabis have to do with the biogenetic pathways of some of the

chemical constituents? What purpose does the resin produced by the secretory glands of the flowering tops and leaves have in the living plant? Is it truly a protection against dry atmosphere and high temperature, or is it in some way concerned physiologically with maturation of the fruit? And why is this resin often produced so much more abundantly by the pistillate plant? What is the purpose to the plant, if any, of the intoxicating constituents found in the resin? How much more study must be placed on the genetics of *Cannabis*! One problem concerns the complexities of sex determination in *Cannabis*, for, while the plant is dioecious, the monoecious condition, which occasionally appears and which has been explained on a genetic basis, can be experimentally induced. Furthermore, sex reversal is still something of a mystery, for plants may occasionally be made to reverse their sex by varying growth conditions. These and many other purely botanical problems await the searchlight of modern research methods.

I trust that, in this brief and admittedly superficial collection of thoughts and queries, I may have awakened in the minds of some of my colleagues in other fields of research germs of ideas which might in some way initiate new chemical and pharmacological research or aid in pursuing older investigations to more productive ends. It is time that one of man's oldest cultivated plants was honoured with the kind of scientific attention that its place in human history and culture merits for it.

Selected References

Adams, R., Marihuana. *Science* 92: 115-119 (1940).

Ames, O., *Economic Annuals and human Cultures.* Botanical Museum of Harvard University, Cambridge, Mass. (1939).

Anonymous, The Cannabis problem: a note on the problem and the history of international action. *Bull. Narcotics* 14, 27-31 (1962).

Bailey, L. H., (Ed.), *Cyclopedia of American Agriculture* 2, 377-380. Macmillan Co., New York, N.Y. (1907).

Bailey, L. H., *The standard Cyclopedia of Horticulture* (2nd Ed.) 1:657-658. Macmillan Co., New York, N.Y. (1942).

Bailey, L. H., *Manual of cultivated Plants* (2nd Ed.) 341. Macmillan Co., New York, N.Y. (1949).

Bailey, L. H. and Bailey, E. Z., *Hortus second* 139-140. 359. Macmillan Co., New York N.Y. (1941).

Bechtel, A. R., The floral anatomy of the Urticales *Amer. Journ. Bot.* 8:386-410 (1921).

Belovitskaia, N. H., *et al., Izv. Akad. Nauk. SSSR Ser. Biol. (Bull. Acad. Sci. URSS. Classe Sci. Math. Nat. Ser Biol.)* 311-334 (1939).

Benson, L., *Plant Classification.* D. C. Heath and Co., Boston, Mass. (1957).

Bentham, G. and Hooker, J. D., *Genera Plantarum* 3:357. L. Reeve and Co., London, England (1880).

Bois, D., *Dictionnaire d'Horticulture* pt. 1 246. Librairie des Sciences Naturelles, Paul Klincksieck, Paris, France (1893-99).

Bouquet, R. J., Cannabis. *Bull. Narcotics* 2, no. 4 (1950) 14-30; 3, no. 1 (1951) 22-43 (1950-51).

Boyce, S. S., *A practical Treatise on the Culture of Hemp (Cannabis sativa) for Seed and Fibre, with a Sketch of the History and Nature of the Plant.* Orange Judd and Co., New York, N.Y. (1900).

Boyce, S. S., *Hemp (Cannabis sativa)* Orange Judd and Co., New York, N.Y. (1912).

Burkill, I. H., *A Dictionary of the economic Products of the Malay Peninsula* 1:437-441. Crown Agents for the Colonies, London, England (1935).

Camp, W. H., The antiquity of hemp as an economic plant. *Journ. New York Bot. Gard.* 37:110-114 (1936).

Charen, S., Facts about marihuana, a survey of the literature. *Amer. Journ. Pharm.* 117:422-430 (1945).

Chopra, I. C. and Chopra, R. N., The use of cannabis drugs in India. *Bull. Narcotics* 9, no. 1:4-29 (1957).

Chopra, R. N., Badhwar, R. L. and Ghosh, S., *Poisonous Plants of India* 2:813-818. Indian Council of Agricultural Research, New Dehli, India (1965).

Cook, O. F., Sexual inequality in hemp. *J. Hered.* 5:203-206 (1914).

Cone, E. L., *Plant Taxonomy* 298. Prentice-Hall Inc., Englewood Cliffs, N.J. (1955).

Cordeiro de Farias, R., Use of maconha *(Cannabis sativa* L.) in Brazil. *Bull. Narcotics* 7, no. 2:5-19 (1955).

Darwin, C., *The Variation of Animals and Plants under·Domestication* 2:201, 331. Orange Judd and Co., New York, N.Y. (1868).

De Candolle, Aug. P., *Prodromus Systematis naturalis Regni vegetabilis* 16, pt. 1:30-31. Treuttel et Wurtz, Paris, France (1824).

De Candolle, Alph. L. P. P., *Géographie botanique raisonée.* 2:833, 981, 986. Librairie de Victor Masson, Geneva, Switzerland (1855).

De Candolle, Alph. L. P. P., *Origin of cultivated Plants.* Kegan Paul, Trench and Co., London, England (1884).

Dewey, L. H., Hemp. *U.S.D.A. Yearbook* 1913:283-346. U.S. Govt. Printing Office, Washington, D.C. (1914).

Dewey, L. H., Hemp varieties of improved type are result of selection. *U.S.D.A. Yearbook of Agriculture* 1927:358-361. U.S. Govt. Printing Office, Washington, D.C. (1928).

Dodge, C. R., A descriptive catalogue of useful fibre plants of the world. *U.S.D.A. Fiber Investigations Rept.* no. 9:106-110. U.S. Govt. Printing Office, Washington, D.C. (1897).

Duquenois, P., Chemical and physiological identification of Indian hemp. *Bull. Narcotics* 2, no. 3:30-33 (1950).

Duthie, J. F. and Fuller, J. B., *Field and garden Crops of the Northwestern Provinces and Oudh, with Illustrations.* Pt. 1:tt. 19, 20, 80-81 (1882). Thomason Civil Eng'g College Press, Roorkie, India.

Eckler, C. R. and Miller, F. A., A study of American grown Cannabis in comparison with samples from various other sources. *Amer. J. Pharm.* 84:488-495 (1912).

Engler, A., *Die natürlichen Pflanzenfamilien* 3, 1:96-98. Wilhelm Engelmann, Leipzig, Germany (1894).

Engler, A., *Syllabus der Pflanzenfamilien* 104-105. Gebruder Borntraeger, Berlin, Germany (1898).

Esau, K., *Plant Anatomy.* John Wiley and Sons, Inc., New York, N.Y. (1953).

Farnsworth, N. R., Hallucinogenic plants. *Science* 162 1086-1092 (1968).

Godwin, H., The ancient cultivation of hemp. *Antiquity* 41:42-50 (1967).

Godwin, H., Pollen analytic evidence for the cultivation of *Cannabis* in England. *Rev. Palaeobot. Palynol.* 4:71-80 (1967).

Grechukhin, E. and Grishko, N., *Comptes Rend. (Docklady) Acad. Sci. USSR* 27:42-46 (1940).

Grlic, L., A comparative study on some chemical and biological characteristics of various samples of Cannabis resin. *Bull. Narcotics* 14, no. 3:37-57 (1962).

Grlic, L., Recent advances in the chemical research of Cannabis. *Bull. Narcotics* 16, no. 4:29-37 (1964).

Gunderson, A., *Families of Dicotyledons,* 138. Chronica Botanica, Waltham, Mass. (1950).

Hamilton, H. C., Cannabis sativa: is the medicinal value found only in the Indian grown drug? *J. Amer. pharm. As.* 4:448-451 (1915).

Hamilton, H. C., The pharmacopoeial requirements for *Cannabis sativa. J. Amer. pharm. Ass.* 1:200-203 (1912).

Hayward, H. E., *The structure of economic Plants.* Macmillan Co., New York., N.Y. (1938).

Hegnauer, R., *Chemotaxonomie der Pflanzen.* 3:350-357. Birkhauser Verlag, Basel, Switzerland (1964).

Heuser, O. (Ed. Herzog, R. O.), Die Hanfpflanze. *Technologie der Textilfasern* 5, pt. 2, *Hanf und Hartfasern,* Julius Springer, Berlin, Germany (1927).

Houghton, E. M. and Hamilton, H. C., A pharmacological study of *Cannabis americana (Cannabis sativa). Amer. J. Pharm.* 80:16-20 (1908).

Huhnke, W. *et al., Zeitschr. f. Pflanzenzucht* 29:55-75 (1950).
Hutchinson, J., *The Families of Flowering Plants* Ed. 2, 1:201. Clarendon Press, Oxford, England (1959).
Joachimoglu, G., Some remarks on the problem of Cannabis *Bull. Narcotics* 11:5-6 (1959).
Johnson, A. M., *Taxonomy of the Flowering Plants,* 202-203. Century Co., New York, N.Y. (1931).
Kabelik, J., Krejci, Z. and Santavy, F., Cannabis as a medicament *Bull. Narcotics* 12, no. 3:5-23 (1960).
Kechatov, E. A., Chemical and biological evaluation of the hemp grown for seed in the central districts of the European part of the USSR. *Bull. Narcotics* 11, no. 4:5-9 (1959).
Lawrence, G. H. M., *Taxonomy of vascular Plants* 463-464. Macmillan Co., New York, N.Y. (1951).
Lemee, A., *Dictionnaire descriptif et synonymique des Genres de Plantes phanerogames* 1:816-817. Imprimerie Commerciale et Administrative, Brest, France (1929).
Lindley, J., *The vegetable Kingdom* 265. Bradbury and Evans, London, England (1847).
Mansfield, R., Vorlaufiges Verzeichnis landwirtschaftlich oder gartnerisch kultivierter Pflanzenarten. *Die Kulturpflanze,* Beih. 2:29-30 (1959).
McGlothlin, W. H., *Hallucinogenic Drugs: a Perspective with special Reference to Peyote and Cannabis* Rand. Corp., Santa Monica, Cal. (1964).
McPhee, H. C., Meiotic cytokinesis of Cannabis. *Bot. Gaz.* 78:335 (1924).
McPhee, H. C., The influence of environment on sex in hemp, *Cannabis sativa* L. *Journ. agric. Res.* 28:1067-1080 (1924).
Morton, J. C., *A Cyclopeida of Agriculture, practical and scientific.* 1:376. Blackie and Son, Glasgow, Scotland (1851).
Murphy, H. B. M., The Cannabis habit. *Bull. Narcotics* 15, pt. 1:15-23 (1963).
Parodi, L. R., *Encyclopedia argentina de Agricultura y Jardineria* 312-314 Editorial Acme S.A.C.I., Buenos Aires, Argentina (1959).
Porter, C. L., *Taxonomy of Flowering Plants* 224-225. W. H. Freeman and Co., San Francisco, Cal. (1959).
Postma, W. P., *Mitosis, meiosis en alloploidie bij Cannabis sativa en Spinacia oleracea.* H. D. Tjeenk Willink en Zoon N.V., Haarlem, Holland. (1946).
Prain, D., *Report on the Cultivation and Use of Ganja.* Bengal Secretariat Press, Calcutta, India (1893).
Pulle, A. A., *Compendium van de Terminologie, Nomenclatuur en Systematiek der Zaadplanten.* Ed. 2 N.V.A. Oosthoek's Uitgevers-Maatschappij, Utrecht, Holland (1950).
Purseglove, J. W., *Tropical Crops. Dicotyledons* 1:40-44. Longmans, Green and Co. Ltd., Harlow, England (1968).

Regallo Pereira, J., Contribução para o estudo das plantas alucinatorias, particularmente da maconha *(Cannabis sativa* L.). *Rev. Fl. Med.* 12:85-209 (1945).

Rendle, A. B., *The classification of Flowering Plants* 2:56-58. Cambridge University Press, Cambridge, England (1959).

Robinson, B. B., Hemp. *Farmers' Bull.* no. 1935, U.S.D.A. U.S. Govt. Printing Office, Washington, D.C. (1943).

Sabalitschka, T., Uber *Cannabis indica,* insbesondere über eine Gewinnung hochwertiger Herba Cannabis Indicae durch Kultur in Deutschland. *Heil- und Gewurz-Pflanzen* 8:73-82 (1925).

Schaffner, J. H., The influence of relative length of day-light on the reversal of sex in hemp. *Ecology* 4:323 (1923).

Schultes, R. E., Hallucinogens of plant origin. *Science* 163:245-254 (1969).

Schwanitz, F., *The Origin of cultivated Plants.* Harvard University Press, Cambridge, Mass. (1966).

Sudell, R., *The new illustrated gardening Encyclopedia* 166, 445. Charles Scribner's Sons, New York, N.Y. (1933).

Synge, P. M. (Ed.), *Royal Horticultural Society, Dictionary of Gardening,* Ed. 2, 1:384. Clarendon Press, Oxford, England (1956).

Talley, P. J., Carbohydrate—nitrogen ratios with respect to the sexual expression of hemp. *Plant Physiol.* 9:731-748 (1934).

Tippo, O., Comparative anatomy of the *Moraceae* and their presumed allies. *Bot. Gaz.* 100:1-99 (1938).

Taylor, N., (Ed.), *Encyclopedia of gardening.* Ed. 2, 165. Houghton, Mifflin Co., Boston, Mass. (1948).

United Nations Economic and Social Council. The possibility of replacing hemp fibre and hemp seed by other crops of similar industrial value or of developing narcotic-free strains of the Cannabis plant. *Commission on Narcotic Drugs,* 10th Session, Item 9. (Mimeographed) (1955).

United States Treasury Department. *Marihuana—its identification.* U.S. Govt. Printing Office, Washington, D.C. (1938).

Vavilov, N. I., *Studies on the Origin of cultivated Plants.* Institute de Botanique Appliquée et d'Amélioration de Plantes, Leningrad, Russia (1926).

Walton, R. P., *Marihuana, America's new drug Problem.* J. P. Lippincott Co., Philadelphia, Penna. (1938).

Watt, G., *Economic Products of India,* pt. 3:13; pt. 4:14 pt. 5:71. Superintendent of Government Printing, Calcutta, India. (1883).

Watt, G., *Dictionary of the economic Products of India* 2: 103-126. Superintendent of Government Printing, Calcutta, India (1889).

Watt, G., *The commercial Products of India*: 249-263. John Murray, London, England (1908).

Watt, J. M. and Breyer-Brandwijk, M. G., *Medicinal and poisonous Plants of southern and eastern Africa.* Ed. 2, 759-772. E. and S. Livingstone Ltd., Edinburgh, Scotland (1962).

Wissett, R., *A Treatise on Hemp*. J. Harding, London, England (1808).

Wollner, H. J., Matchett, J. R., Levine, J. and Valaer, P., Report of the marihuana investigation. *J. Amer. pharm. Ass.* 27:29-36 (1938).

Zhukovskii, P. M., *Cultivated Plants and their wild Relatives (Systematics, Geography, Cytogenetics, Ecology, Origin)* Ed. 2 Koios, Leningrad, Russia (1964).

Zhukovskii, P. M., *Cultivated Plants and their wild Relatives* (transl. P. S. Hudson) Commonwealth Agricultural Bureau, Farnham Royal, Bucks., England (1962).

3 Some Ecological Implications of the Distribution of Hemp (*Cannabis sativa L.*) in the United States of America*

Alan Haney and Fakhri A. Bazzaz

Hemp may be one of the most widely distributed plants. Probably native to Asia, hemp is now spread throughout most of the temperate and tropic regions of the world. The species attains good growth at 7,000 feet in the Himalaya Mountains (Royle, 1855); it exists widely in tropical Africa, East Africa, and South Africa (Watt and Breyer-Brandwijk, 1962) as well as Hawaii (Tutin *et al.,* 1964). The species was apparently introduced into the United States by the pilgrims as early as 1632 (Dewey, 1913); it now occurs from Quebec to British Columbia in Canada and south throughout the United States (Muencher, 1955).

Hemp is usually described as a tall, robust, annual herb (Pratt and Youngken, 1951); however, the size and vigour vary widely depending on the site. The species is dioecious; the ratio of male to female plants is reportedly influenced by exposure of seeds to ultra-violet light (Montemartini, 1926), by day-length (Schaffner, 1923, 1931), by air temperature (Cheuvart, 1954), by carbon monoxide concentration (Heslop-Harrison, 1957), by the age of pollen and the stigma (Laskowska, 1961), and by the nitrogen concentration in the soil solution (Arnoux, 1966a, 1966b).

Ecological information on seeds and seed germination of wild hemp is sparse. Most studies have been directed to commercial management or to the physiology of the species. Besides the studies

* The authors wish to acknowledge the assistance of Benjamin Kutscheid in summarizing the data.

39

noted above, Wilsie and Reddy (1946) studied seed treatment and Jordan *et al.* (1946), Wilsie *et al.* (1944), and Black and Vessel (1945) examined response of the species to soil fertilization. Effects of storage treatment on hemp seeds and germination stimulation were studied by Malinovskii (1927), Stephan (1928), Dorywalski (1935), Koehler (1946), and Suput (1954). Dewey (1913) noted that hemp germinated best when planted 1.25 cm below the surface.

Man has undoubtedly been the major disseminator of hemp seeds on the regional scale. Locally, birds are probably the most important feeders on hemp seeds and may be important in its spread. Hanson and Kossack (1963) found small amounts of hemp seeds in the crops of mourning doves in south central Illinois; however, hemp was by far the most important food of doves in southwest Iowa (McClure, 1943). Pheasants are expected to feed heavily on hemp seeds, but because they are not migratory, they would only be important in local spread.

Hemp for fibre production is reported to grow best on well-drained, friable soils that are high in nitrogen and organic matter (Dewey, 1913). Barnyard manure was often used as a fertilizer for hemp. Royle (1855) reported that the cooler the soil, the more manure was required to produce good fibre yields. These observations suggest that in cooler areas hemp may be more restricted to sites high in nitrogen or organic matter. Goss (1924) reported no hemp germination after one to 24 years storage of seeds in the soil. This suggests that hemp seeds are not long-lived in the soil, but further studies are needed.

Apparently on the basis of fibre yields, hemp was reported to be susceptible to drought (Hackleman and Domingo, 1943). Numerous specimens of hemp, however, have been collected from sandy soils in Illinois, including a sand prairie in the west-central part of the state. Many of these specimens were flowering or fruiting, although most were less than one metre tall. This indicates that the species may be physiologically able to tolerate dry sites, although fibre production obviously would be very low. Early frost may bring about premature death of hemp in the autumn (Dewey, 1913) and young plants are easily injured by frost (Royle, 1855). The plant is reported to invade and become established on disturbed sites quickly, particularly if early weed growth is restricted. Once hemp is growing well, it is believed to control competing weeds, especially annuals (Hackleman and Domingo, 1943). Royle (1855) simply stated, "Hemp will smother all weeds". Although weed control by hemp was believed to result from shading by the fast growing annual, another mechanism may be operative. Pratt and Youngken (1951) reported that hemp produced volatile oils comprised of terpenes and sesquiterpenes. Most terpenes inhibit germination and growth at high concentrations. For example, Muller *et al.* (1964), and Muller and Hauge (1967), found that a western shrub, *Salvia leucophylla,* produced volatile terpenes that greatly restricted the growth of annual grasses. Since hemp seedlings contain little of the narcotic principle (Kingsbury, 1964), the volatile oils, also, may not be produced until the plant is well established. The inability of young hemp to control weed competition, mentioned by Hackleman and Domingo, may simply reflect the lack of development of terpene production.

Dewey (1913) reported few isolated instances of fungus diseases killing hemp. In each case, the hemp was growing in an unfavourable site, had been damaged by hail, or was planted late in the spring. Few animals browse hemp and few insects attack the species in the United States. Although a fungus may attack seeds and reduce germination, Robinson (1943) reported that hemp seedlings are remarkably free of seedling diseases. Dewey (1913) noted that a root parasite, branched broom rape (*Orobanche ramosa*), a European species of only scattered occurrence in the United States, was the only serious enemy to cultivated hemp. Where it was abundant, the broom rape killed large numbers of hemp plants before they flowered. Broom rape might conceivably be a natural control of hemp, but research is needed to determine how effective this would be and whether other, more desirable, plant species would suffer from the spread. This species of broom rape has been reported to attack tobacco and tomato.

Before starting an intensive study of the ecology of hemp, we have attempted to review and summarize existing information. Much information can be obtained by a review of botanical specimens of the species in the herbaria. We have summarized the data contained on about 1,600 hemp specimens from 86 of the major herbaria in the United States. These data include date and location from which the specimens were collected, sex, and usually, site remarks. From these data, we have obtained many suggestions regarding the ecology of hemp.

The rate of establishment of newly introduced species usually follows

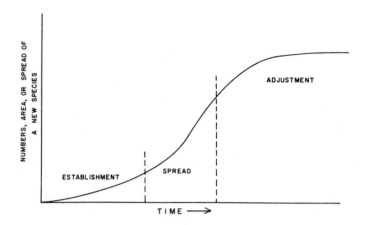

Fig. 1. The normal pattern of spread of a new species in a defined area.

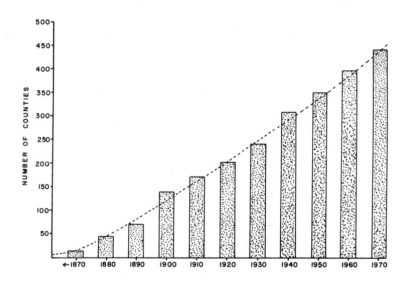

Fig. 2. Number of counties in the United States of America from which hemp was collected by the date indicated (number for 1970 extrapolated).

the normal "S-shaped" growth curve (Fig. 1). The actual rate of expansion of any species in a new range will depend on the species and its suitability to the range. The species may rapidly spread to some sites and require years before becoming established in others. As recently as 1943, Hackleman and Domingo reported that there was little need to fear the escape and spread of hemp. However, hemp is now extremely widespread in the Midwest of the United States and occurs in most major cities of the country, except those in the South. Collection of botanical specimens of hemp reflect the spread. Figure 2, based on the numbers of counties in the United

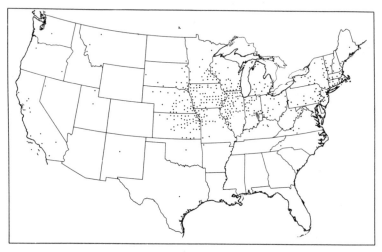

Fig. 3. Distribution of hemp by United States of America counties. A dot indicates that an escaped specimen was collected at least once in the county.

States where hemp has been collected, shows the slowly accelerating spread of the species. Although it is difficult from these data to decide where on the model of growth hemp is now, there is no indication that it is in the adjustment phase.

Several general trends in the distribution of hemp in the United States, based on collected specimens, are of interest (Fig. 3). Only in certain sections of the Midwest is the species widespread and abundant. It is very common in the East, but seldom achieves the lush stands common in Iowa, Illinois and Missouri. The species is not at all common in the dry or mountainous regions of the West, and its occurrence is usually scattered, isolated colonies, most often in cities. The variety of hemp present in the United States has almost certainly escaped from crop plants grown for fibre or oil. This variety was imported from the cool, temperate areas of Europe or Asia. Apparently, this variety does not grow in the warmer regions as evidenced by the distinct absence of the species in the southern United States. Finally, there is a good correlation of hemp distribution with alluvial soils along streams. This trend is most apparent in Missouri, Kansas, Nebraska, Iowa, Minnesota and South Dakota. Alluvial sites usually have soil conditions well suited to the species, they are frequently disturbed by flooding, and seeds of hemp may be carried in flood water.

A closer examination of hemp distribution in Illinois reveals an interesting pattern (Fig. 4). The species is virtually nonexistent in the southeastern portion of the state. It is also absent or very sparse in a large area in the northeastern section. A common characteristic of these areas is a tight soil high in clay. The southern part of the state is low in nitrogen. (Recall that hemp was reported to do poorly on soils low in nitrogen or high in clay.) Lack of clay is probably more important in hemp establishment since numerous specimens of hemp have been collected in very sandy soils that are extremely low in nitrogen. Specimens from these sites are generally small, but they persist and produce fruits. Seldom, however, have hemp plants been collected from soils high in clay.

One other interesting result has come from this preliminary study of hemp specimens in the United States. Of the 1,404 plants the sex of which was reported, 55 per cent were male. However, of the 248 specimens collected from along streets and highways, only 41 per cent were male. Thus, an unexpectedly low percentage of hemp plants along roads was male. The probability of this difference resulting from chance is less than one per cent. Heslop-Harrison (1957) demonstrated that exposure of hemp plants to low levels of CO for brief periods of time would cause a shift in sex expression from male to female. This is a possible explanation for the higher proportion of female plants along roads. Ecologically, the increase in ratio of female plants is important. Because hemp is wind pollinated, one male plant probably produces sufficient pollen to fertilize flowers on more than one female plant. A relative increase in the number of female plants would result in more seeds. The evolutionary advantage of a device for increasing the ratio of female to male plants on dioecious species becomes apparent.

Hemp is already a major problem in the United States as a source

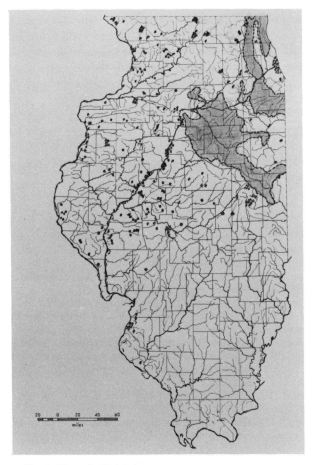

Fig. 4. Places in Illinois where hemp specimens have been collected. Darkened areas are regions of soils high in clay.

of marijuana. Although the variety present throughout most of the country is reportedly low in narcotic derivatives, it is still widely collected and used. Evidence from this study suggests that hemp is spreading in the United States at an increasing rate. Spread is most rapid in the Midwest on alluvial soils and soils relatively low in clay; however, the species can and does invade sites less suited. It shows a tremendous ecological amplitude in this respect and has been collected in nearly every conceivable site from lake shores to cracks in concrete walls and upland pine plantations. Although most of the marijuana used in the United States at present results from imported material, as that source is controlled the naturalized variety will probably be used much more. Controlling the collection of a weed that occurs in thousands of vacant lots across the country will be a problem of tremendous magnitude.

Although our study of the ecology of hemp is just beginning, we already have indications of some very interesting problems. Solution to many of these problems may help our understanding of some basic problems in population biology, plant geography, and plant ecology.

References

Arnoux, M., Influence des facteurs du millieu sur l'expression de la sexualité du chanvre monoïque (*Cannabis sativa* L.). *Ann. Amélior Plantes* 16(3):259-262 (1966a).

Arnoux, M., Influence des facteurs du millieu sur l'expression de la sexualité du chanvre monoïque (*Cannabis sativa* L.): II. Action de la nutrition azotée. *Ann. Amélior Plantes* 16(2):123-134 (1966b).

Black, C. A. and Vessel, A. J., The response of hemp to fertilizers in Iowa. *Soil Sci. Soc. Amer. Proc.* 9:178-184 (1945).

Cheuvart, C., Studies on the development of *Cannabis sativa* L. at constant temperature and under different photoperiods (sexuality and foliage pigments). *Bull. Acad. Roy. Med. Belg.: C. Science* 40:1152-1168 (1954).

Dewey, L. H., Hemp. In: *Yearbook of the U.S. Dept. of Agric.* 1913, pp. 283-346 (1913).

Dorywalski, J., The cooperation of external agents in germination. *Roezniki Nauk Rolniczych Lesnych* 35:79-140 (1935). (Cited from *Biol. Abstr.* 10:15443 (1936).)

Goss, W. L., The viability of buried seeds. *J. Agr. Res.* 29:349-362 (1924).

Hackleman, J. C. and Domingo, W. E., Hemp, an Illinois war crop. *Univ. of Ill. Agr. Exp. Sta., Cir.* No. 547. (1943).

Hanson, H. C. and Kossack, C. W., The mourning dove in Illinois. *Ill. Dept. Cons. Tech. Bull.* No. 2 (1963).

Heslop-Harrison, J., The experimental modification of sex expression in flowering plants. *Biol. Rev.* 32:1-51 (1957).

Jordon, H. V., Lang, A. L. and Enfield, G. H., Effects of fertilizers on yields and breaking strengths of American hemp, *Cannabis sativa*. *J. Amer. Soc. Agron.* 38:551-563 (1946).

Kingsbury, John M., *Poisonous plants of the United States and Canada*. Prentice-Hall, Inc., Englewood Cliffs, N.J. (1964).

Koehler, B., Hemp seed treatments in relation to different dosages and conditions of storage. *Phytopath.* 36:937-942 (1946).

Laskowska, R., Influence of the age of pollen and stigmas on sex determination in hemp. *Nature* 192:147-148 (1961).

Malinovskii, S. M., Stimulation of hemp seed (*Cannabis sativa* L.). *Mem. Inst. Agron. a'Lenin* 4:289-348 (1927). (Cited from *Biol. Abstr.* 4:23899 (1930).)

McClure, H. E., Ecology and management of the mourning dove, *Zenaidura macroura* (Linn.), in Cass County, Iowa. *Iowa Agr. Exp. Sta. Res. Bull.* 310:355-415 (1943).

Montemartini, Luigi, Effetti del trattamento del polline col metodo Pirovano sopra la proporzione dei sessi nella *Cannabis sativa* L. *Rend. R. Ist. Lombardo* 2 Ser. 59:748-752 (1926). (Cited from *Biol. Abstr.* 2:9577 (1928).)

Muencher, W. C., *Weeds*. Macmillian, New York, N.Y. (1955).

Muller, W. H. and Hauge, R., Volatile growth inhibitors produced by *Salvia leucophylla:* effect on seedling anatomy. *Bull. Torrey Bot. Club* 94:182-190 (1967).

Muller, C. H., Muller, W. H. and Haines, B. L., Volatile growth inhibitors produced by aromatic shrubs. *Science* 143:471-473 (1964).

Pratt, R. and H. W. Youngken, Jr., *Pharmacognosy*. J. B. Lippincott Co., Philadelphia, Penna. (1951).

Robbins, W. W., Bellue, M. K. and Ball, W. S., *Weeds of California*. Sta. Dept. Agr., Sacramento, Calif. (1941).

Robinson, B. B., Greenhouse seed treatment studies on hemp. *J. Amer. Soc. Agron.* 35:910 (1943).

Royle, J. F., *Fibrous plants of India*. Smith, Elder, and Co., London. (1855).

Schaffner, J. H., The influence of relative length of daylight on the reversal of sex in hemp. *Ecology* 4:323-334 (1923).

Schaffner, J. H., The functional curve of sex-reversal in staminate hemp plants induced by photoperiodicity. *Amer. J. Bot.* 18:424-430 (1931).

Stephan, J., Stimulationversuche mit *Cannabis sativa. Faser frosch.* 7:292-298 (1928). (Cited from *Biol. Abstr.* 6:6636 (1932).)

Suput, M., The effect of soil moisture on germination and growth of sowing of soybeans, vetch, sunflower, flax, hemp and turnip. *Zbornik Radova Belgrade Univ. Poljoprivrendi* Fok. 2:68-80 (1954). (*Soil Fertilizers* 18:219 (1955).)

Tutin, T. G., Heywood, V. H., Burges, N. A., Valentine, D. H., Walters, S. M. and Webb, D. A., *Flora Europaea. Vol. 1*.

Lycopodiaceae to Platanaceae. Cambridge University Press. (1964).

Watt, J. M. and Breyer-Brandwijk, M. G., *The medicinal and poisonous plants of southern and eastern Africa.* E. and S. Livingstone, London (1962).

Wilsie, C. R., Black, C. A. and Aandahl, A. R., Hemp production experiments, cultural practices and soil requirements. *Iowa Agr. Exp. Sta. and Iowa Sta. Col. Agr. Ext. Serv. Comp. Bull.* p. 63 (1944).

Wilsie, C. P. and Reddy, C. S., Seed treatment experiments with hemp. *J. Amer. Soc. Agron.* 38:693-701 (1946).

4 Changes with Maturation in the Amounts of Biologically Interesting Substances of Cannabis

Zdeněk Krejčí

There are still many problems concerning hashish. Even now it is difficult to discover the substances in Cannabis responsible for the effect of hashish; or ways of objectively estimating the narcotic effects; or the mechanism of the effect of these substances on the organism; or what metabolites occur after Cannabis use; how they can be demonstrated in biological fluids, etc. There is no general agreement about the conditions necessary for the production of the substances with hashish effect in the plant. Another significant question is closely connected with this one. *Cannabis sativa,* cultivated in a mild climate for industrial use, contains biologically active substances: to what extent does development of the narcotic principle parallel the antibiotic activity? Neither is it known at what degree of maturation of the plant natural biosynthesis of the hashish principle occurs.

The structure of some substances in Cannabis is remarkably similar, although their pharmacological effect is so different. Some years ago, the striking coincidence of these chemical structures gave rise to the idea that those substances represent various stages of biosynthesis. We demonstrated that substances with antibiotic activity from *Cannabis indica* are not identical with the substance or complex responsible for the hashish effect. Our opinion, which is in harmony with that of other groups, is that the antibiotically effective substances of hemp are forerunners of substances of cannabinol type, and that these change at full ripeness under optimal conditions,

49

especially of temperature, to the tetrahydrocannabinol with the hashish effect.

This study is a contribution to the solution of this complex and fundamental problem.

During three seasons (1964-66) *Cannabis sativa* was cultivated in the temperate climate of Czechoslovakia. Cultures from two localities were examined systematically at weekly intervals from the age of 4 weeks (height 25 cm) until full ripeness, i.e. 21 weeks (250 cm high). Attention was paid to the conditions of cultivation as well as to climatic and meteorological conditions. *Cannabis sativa* of the Rastislav variety, specially improved for the industrial production of fibres in Czechoslovakia, was used. Two localities with very different soil characteristics were chosen. Locality I was very well prepared with fertilized soil, and locality II had a poor and unmanured soil.

Homogenous samples of the drug, obtained by crushing and mixing at least ten female plants, were used. At the earlier stages, when the height of individual plants did not reach 1 m, whole plants were used; later the sample was obtained by mixing and homogenizing ten plant tops, 1 metre long, to eliminate the strong, relatively heavy and leafless stalks, poor in resinous substances, which would have substantially distorted the results.

Extractions were made with ethyl alcohol and, in parallel, with petroleum ether from the homogenous samples of the fresh material. After concentrating these in a vacuum, the percentage amount of extractable substances was determined.

In the next stage we quantitatively isolated the biologically active amorphous resin (IRC) by shaking these extracts with NaOH solution.

The extracts so prepared and the isolated resin fractions were analysed by ascending thin-layer chromatography. Spots were detected by bi-diazotized benzidine, followed by 3, 4 dibromchinonchlorimid. New spots, i.e. new substances, successively appeared at different stages of the plants' development. Their relations to the appearance and growth of antibiotic activity were also studied.

In parallel with these analyses, we examined the growth of antibiotic activity in freshly pressed sap, in all standard concentrated extracts and the above-mentioned isolated resin fractions, at 1% concentration in chloroform. The antibiotic effect was determined by cultivation, on a solid culture medium by the modified Oxford method, of the standard B *subtilis* microorganism.

The target of this part of the research was to find the stage of development and degree of ripeness of the plant at which new spots appeared on the chromatogram. These substances were compared chromatographically with standard cannabidiolic acid, cannabidiol and tetrahydrocannabinol solutions.

RESULTS

(a) Influence of the quality of the soil upon plant growth

The expected, relatively large difference in plant height between the two groups, and the delayed growth in locality II were observed

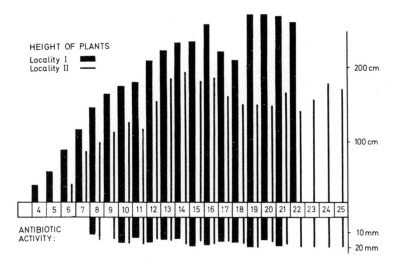

Fig. 1. Height and potency of Cannabis plants grown in two localities.

(Fig. 1). The delay of approximately three or four weeks became especially evident in the first third of the growing season. While the cultures from locality I reached the stage of full ripeness at 250 cm, the plants from locality II were weak and on average 1 m shorter. This fact demonstrated to us that we had indeed created different experimental conditions.

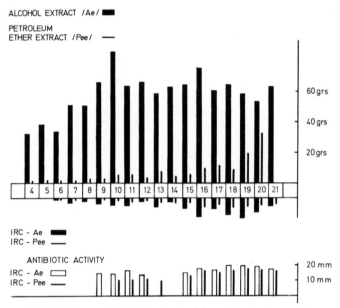

Fig. 2. Potency of various extracts of Cannabis plants grown in locality I.

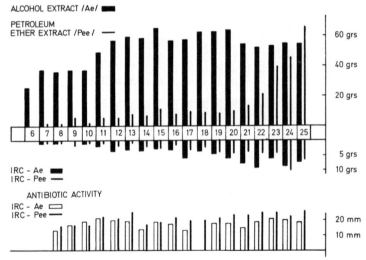

Fig. 3. Potency of various extracts of Cannabis plants grown in locality II.

(b) Antibiotic activity at different degrees of ripeness

Antibiotic activity was found in plants from both localities from the eighth week onwards (Fig. 1). Paradoxically, it appeared that, especially in the initial phase, the activity was greater in cultures from locality II, i.e. from the worse conditions of cultivation. This was subsequently confirmed (Figs. 2 and 3).

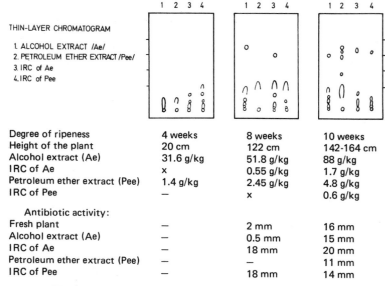

THIN-LAYER CHROMATOGRAM

1. ALCOHOL EXTRACT /Ae/
2. PETROLEUM ETHER EXTRACT /Pee/
3. IRC of Ae
4. IRC of Pee

Degree of ripeness	4 weeks	8 weeks	10 weeks
Height of the plant	20 cm	122 cm	142-164 cm
Alcohol extract (Ae)	31.6 g/kg	51.8 g/kg	88 g/kg
IRC of Ae	x	0.55 g/kg	1.7 g/kg
Petroleum ether extract (Pee)	1.4 g/kg	2.45 g/kg	4.8 g/kg
IRC of Pee	—	x	0.6 g/kg
Antibiotic activity:			
Fresh plant	—	2 mm	16 mm
Alcohol extract (Ae)	—	0.5 mm	15 mm
IRC of Ae	—	18 mm	20 mm
Petroleum ether extract (Pee)	—	—	11 mm
IRC of Pee	—	18 mm	14 mm

Fig. 4. Thin layer chromatograms of various extracts of Cannabis plants grown in locality I.

(c) Amount of alcohol and petroleum ether soluble material at different stages of development

We were not surprised by the high extractive ability of alcohol (Figs. 2 and 3) but by the relatively low extractive power of petroleum ether, especially in the early stages of plant development. A change in favour of petroleum ether occurs in the later stages of full development, when it is much more advantageous to use petroleum ether. The same is true in relation to IRC, especially at the earlier stages. The amount of IRC obtained by petroleum ether extraction is significantly lower than that by alcohol extraction.

However, the quality of IRC obtained by both methods of
extraction does not differ in regard to antibiotic activity. In the
fresh material IRC quality varies slightly from ten weeks until full
ripeness (Fig. 2). There was no essential difference in the amounts of
extracted material from the two localities at any stage of development. Quantitatively, locality II, i.e. that with worse soil, was
slightly superior.

(d) Estimation of different stages of development of Cannabis by thin-layer chromatography

The alcohol and petroleum ether extracts were concentrated to
half volume: 1% solutions of IRC were prepared in chloroform.

Representative chromatograms at several important stages of
development show changes with maturation in relation to other
physico-chemical and microbiological factors (Fig. 4). With sufficient
numbers of acceptable comparative standards, the beginnings of
answers to a number of the questions mentioned at the beginning
can be attempted.

CONCLUSION

It has been confirmed that cannabidiolic acid appears at relatively
early stages of development. Increasing amounts are found, especially
in fresh material, at all further degrees of development until full
ripeness. In dried material especially if stored for a long time, the
amount of cannabidiolic acid decreases as a result of decarboxylation
and evidently changes to cannabidiol. Cannabidiolic acid is known to
have antibiotic activity, which may account for the parallel between
the appearance of cannabidiolic acid and that of antibiotic activity
traced from the eighth week of development.

The influence of the quality of the soil upon the growth and
quantity of active substances developed is very interesting. The
quality of the soil positively influences the growth and height of
plants, but has no perceptible effect upon the production of extractable substances. The amount of IRC and antibiotic activity produced
from less fertile localities is greater. The changes that occur in different stages of development are accompanied by large changes in the
quantity of substances extractable by alcohol and petroleum ether.
The increase in the amount extractable in petroleum ether at later

stages of development is especially noteworthy. These observations confirm the occurrence of qualitative changes in the chemical structure of plant constituents.

Pharmacological evaluation on experimental animals will follow the physicochemical results reported here, and will be the subject of further communications.

5 Constituents of Male and Female Cannabis

Stig Agurell

with the participation of Inger Nilsson, J. Lars, G. Nilsson, Agneta
Ohlsson, Kerstin Olofsson, Finn Sandberg and Marianne Wahlqvist
of the Faculty of Pharmacy and Jan-Erik Lindgren of the Department
of Toxicology, Karolinska Institute Stockholm.

According to present data (Schultz and Hoffner, 1960; Claussen and
Korte, 1968), previous suggestions (Mechoulam and Gaoni, 1965;
Grlic, 1964) implying biosynthesis of cannabidiolic and tetrahydrocannabinolic acid from a monoterpene residue (geraniol pyrophos-
phate) and olivetolic acid seems probable. Possibly, cannabigerolic
acid may be the first condensation product. The "primer" for the
formation of olivetolic acid would apparently be hexanoate, which
in turn is condensed with three acetate units yielding olivetolic acid.
Biochemical analogies to this reaction are known. The ability of
different Cannabis strains to produce either mainly cannabidiolic
acid or tetrahydrocannabinolic acid is genetically determined. But
it is also well known that climatic factors and the stage of plant
development are of considerable importance and particularly so for
further secondary transformations of the Cannabis constituents.

As pointed out in a recent paper by Valle, Lapa and Barros (1968),
there is a general belief that only female plants of *Cannabis sativa*
contain the active ingredients of Cannabis preparations (hashish,
marihuana). They investigated resin from male and female Cannabis
using pharmacological tests and concluded that male and female
plants exhibited similar pharmacological activity.

We have qualitatively and quantitatively compared the chemical
constituents of male and female Cannabis by gas and thin-layer
chromatography as well as mass spectrometry. *Cannabis sativa*
obtained from Jugoslavia was grown in a green-house and the flowering

57

male and female plants were collected separately. Four different
parts of each sex were compared: (a) flowers; (b) upper leaves (sur-
rounding the flowers); (c) large leaves (from lower part of the stem);
(d) stems (lower part). Fresh plant material was extracted with
methylene chloride as described by Claussen and Korte (1968). The
extracts were chromatographed (Agurell, Nilsson, Ohlsson and
Sandberg, 1969; Korte and Sieper, 1964) by GLC (5% SE-30 on Gas

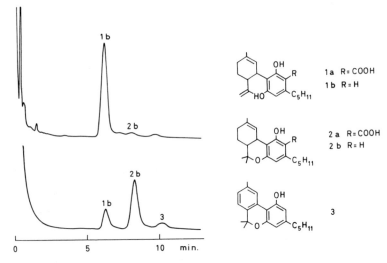

Fig. 1. Gas chromatographic separation of cannabinoid constituents of: (upper panel) flowers of male *Cannabis sativa:*
and, (lower panel) extract of a hashish preparation. Cannabidiolic
acid (*1a*), cannabidiol (*1b*), Δ1-tetrahydrocannabinolic acid
(*2a*), Δ1-tetrahydrocannabinol (*2b*), cannabinol (*3*).

Chrom P; 6 ft. x 1/8 in. glass column; 220°; Aerograph 204) and
TLC (formamide-impregnated silica gel G using 20% ether in light
petroleum solvent system; spray reagent, Echtblausalz). Native
extracts as well as diazomethane treated extracts, in which acids
were converted to methyl esters, were compared with reference
compounds. Identification was also carried out by combined gas
chromatography—mass spectrometry (GLC-MS) (Agurell, Holmstedt,
Lindgren and Schultes, 1969). Cannabidiolic acid (*1a*) partly decarboxylated in the gas chromatograph to yield cannabidiol (*1b*), which
was identified by GLC-MS.

In agreement with previous investigators we found the European hemp investigated (Fig. 1). to contain cannabidiolic acid (*1a*) as the main cannabinol of fresh hemp (over 95%) with minor amounts (3%) of apparently Δ^1-tetrahydrocannabinolic acid (*2a*). The same compounds, although to some degree decarboxylated, were present in plants grown from the same seed lot in Jugoslavia.

TABLE 1. *Content of cannabinols of male and female hemp**

	Mg/g fresh weight	
Plant part	Male	Female
Flowers	0.88	1.86
Upper leaves	2.75	2.30
Large Leaves	0.85	0.96
Stem	0.34	0.12

* Estimated as cannabidiol

Qualitative comparison of different sexes and parts showed the same compounds in similar ratios. The quantitative estimate of cannabinols established that the male and female plants contain similar amounts of cannabinols per fresh weight of plant material. However, the mature female plants have richer foliage and consequently yield more cannabinols per plant than the slender male plants.

Incorporation experiments with these plants in the summer of 1968 with radioactive precursors (acetate, hexanoate, mevalonate, geraniol) failed to yield any radioactive cannabinols. Possibly the precursors were administered too late in the season when all the cannabinols had already been formed.

References

Agurell, S., Holmstedt, B., Lindgren, J. E. and Schultes, R. E., *Acta. chem. Scand.* 23:903 (1969).

Agurell, S., Nilsson, I. M., Ohlsson, A. and Sandberg, F., *Biochem. Pharmacol.* 18:1195 (1969).

Claussen, U. and Korte, F., *Ann.* 713:162 (1968).

Claussen, U. and Korte, F., *Ann.* 713:166 (1968).

Grlic, L., *Bull. Narcotics.* 16, No. 4, 29 (1964).

Korte, F. and Sieper, H., *J. Chromatog.* 13:90 (1964).

Mechoulam, R. and Gaoni, Y., *Tetrahedron* 21:1223 (1965).

Schultz, O. E. and Hoffner, G., *Arch. Pharm.* 293:1 (1960).

Valle, J. R., Lapa, A. J. and Barros, G. G., *J. Pharm. Pharmac.* 20:798 (1968).

6 Microscopic Detection of Cannabis in the Pure State and in Semi-Combusted Residues

Arnold Nordal

My contact with cannabis problems and my experience in this field is mainly based on cooperation with the Police Department of Oslo, for which institution I have been a consultant in narcotic matters for several years.

When samples of plant materials seized by the police are handed over for analysis, they are often accompanied by a standard question: "Does this sample contain cannabis?"

Very often the samples are brought in by a policeman, who comes from the airport and presses for an answer while his car is waiting outside.

In these and similar cases where a quick answer is demanded, the microscopic method is the simplest. But this method is also a very useful tool in the detection of cannabis and cannabis preparations intended for or used for smoking. (I would like to point out that there are many cases where the microscopic method can at the most only provide certain indications, and where other methods, like thin layer chromatography, might give a far more dependable answer.)

The basis for a reliable microscopic method is that the plant material in question has characteristic histological elements (trichomes, crystals etc.) that can be used as guiding principles in the analysis.

Fortunately, cannabis has a very characteristic anatomical structure. This is especially true for the flowering and fruiting tops of the plant, which, according to the "Single Convention on Narcotic Drugs 1961", make up the narcotic drug.

A short survey follows of the micromorphological elements from the flowering or fruiting tops of the plant, of the cannabis resin and of microscopic semi-combusted fragments that remain in pipes used for smoking cannabis.

THE FLOWERING OR FRUITING TOPS (= MARIHUANA)

Figure 1 shows a fruiting top of the plant and material derived from it. Most of the marihuana samples that I have examined have contained ripe or nearly ripe fruits. To reach this state of development, the plant must be about 6-8 months old. A growing season of this length is found only in the tropics. In a cold climate, like that of Norway, the growing season is only 4-5 months, by which time few plants have yet started to develop flowers at all (see below).

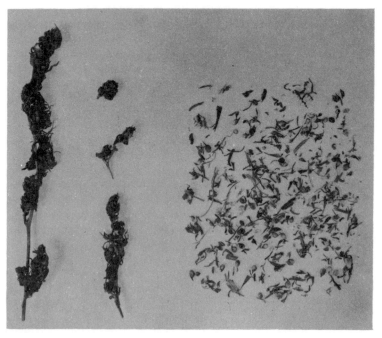

Fig. 1. Fruiting top and material derived from it.

For the microscopic detection of marihuana, the numerous bracts found in the flowering and fruiting tops of the cannabis plants are of special interest.

These bracts show a dorsiventral structure (Fig. 2). The palisade

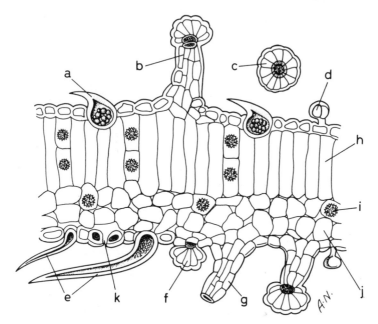

Fig. 2. Cross section of a bract from the fruiting plant.

(a) Cystolith hair
(b) Large glandular hair with several cells in head and stalk
(c) Head of one of the large glandular hairs
(d) small glandular hair with bicellular head and unicellular stalk
(e) Thick walled conical trichomes
(f) Large developing glandular hair
(g) Stalk of a large glandular hair
(h) Palisade cell
(i) Cluster crystal

usually consists of a single layer, rarely two, of cylindrical cells, and the spongy tissue of two to four layers of rounded parenchyma. Cluster crystals of calcium oxalate are present in all parts of the mesophyll. The upper epidermis bears unicellular, sharply pointed, curved conical trichomes, about 150-220 μ long, with enlarged bases

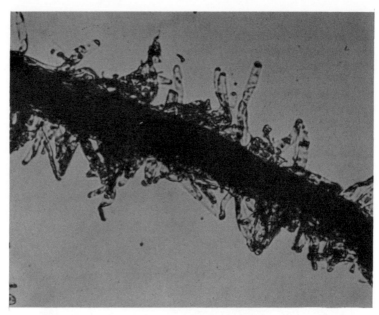

Fig. 3. Fragment of stigma.

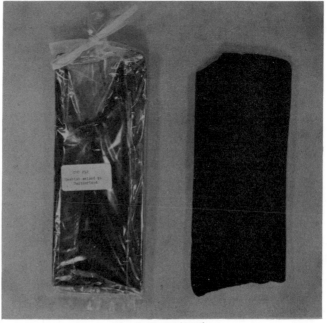

Fig. 4. Cannabis resin.

in which there are cystoliths of calcium carbonate. In the upper epidermis numerous glandular trichomes are also found with a secreting head of about eight radiating club-shaped cells.

Some of these glands are sessile and others have a cylindrical, multicellular stalk, about 200 μ long and several cells in diameter. The lower epidermis bears conical trichomes which are longer than those of the upper side (about 340 to 500 μ long) and more slender, but without cystoliths. Small glandular hairs with a bicellular head and unicellular stalk are found on both sides of the bracts. Stomata are present on the under surface, but are absent from the upper surface.

The glands and the cystolith hairs are the most important guiding principles for the microscopic detection both of marihuana and cannabis resin.

The dark brown and forked stigmas or fragments thereof are often found in samples of marihuana or hashish. Nearly every epidermis cell of the stigmas is extended as a unicellular papilla about 90 to 180 μ long with a rounded apex (Fig. 3).

CANNABIS RESIN (= HASHISH)

Figure 4 shows two samples of cannabis resin. To the left a plate of resin (24 x 9 x 0.8 cm) wrapped in plastic, and to the right an unwrapped plate. The samples were put at my disposal by Dr. Olav Braenden, Director of the United Nations Narcotics Laboratory, Geneva.

Figure 5 shows a microscopic preparation of cannabis resin with the different types of trichomes shown in Fig. 2 (hairs with cystoliths, stalks and heads of glandular hairs, conical trichomes etc.). A significant part of the so-called cannabis resin is made up of these trichomes.

SEMI-COMBUSTED RESIDUES FROM PIPES USED FOR SMOKING CANNABIS

When cannabis or cannabis resin is smoked in pipes, the heads of the glands with their high oily or resinous content are first attacked. Then follow the stalks of the same trichomes together with the soft parenchyma of the bracts.

The most persistent parts are the conical trichomes from the lower epidermis of the bracts (cp. Fig. 6). As a rule the more thin-walled basic parts of these trichomes disappear first, while the thick-

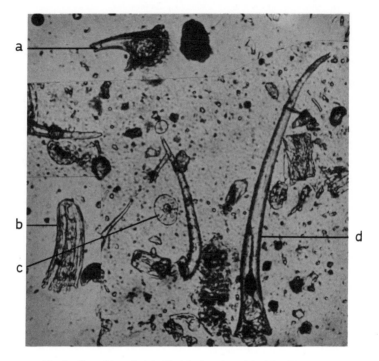

Fig. 5. Cannabis resin (clarified by heating with chloral hydrate)
   (a) Cystolith hair
   (b) Stalk of large glandular hair
   (c) Head of large glandular hair
   (d) Large conical hair from lower epidermis with thin-walled
       base.

walled upper parts show a very high power of resistance. Semi-combusted fragments of these trichomes are therefore of great importance in the microscopic examination of pipes used for smoking cannabis.

ADMIXTURES OF TOBACCO LEAVES

The pipes that are used for smoking cannabis are often used for smoking tobacco. This should be kept in mind when examining pipes seized by persons suspected of cannabis smoking.

   Fragments of tobacco leaves are easy to recognize because of their characteristic trichomes of different types, and even more,

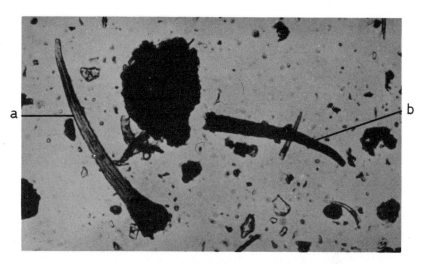

Fig. 6. Semi-combusted residues from pipes used for smoking cannabis resin.

(a) Large conical trichome with semi-combusted base
(b) Semi-combusted top of a corresponding hair.

because of their rounded idioblasts containing sandy microsphenoidal crystals of calcium oxalate.

I should like to add a few words about a cannabis cultivation project started in Norway last summer, a small part of a bigger project organized by Dr. Olav Braenden, to study the influence of ecological factors on the morphology and chemistry of the cannabis plant.

We used three types of seeds of *Cannabis sativa:* one of Swiss origin, one of Lebanese origin and the third from South Africa. The seeds were planted at the same time in three localities: one in Oslo (60°N), one in the middle of Norway, and one north of the arctic circle (69°N).

The seeds were planted in the middle of May and the plants harvested in the middle of September, so the growing season was about 4 months.

The plants of the three localities showed an astonishingly parallel rate of development. There were clear differences in the plants originating from the three types of seeds, but the individual plants of the three origins were very similar in their height, branching and micromorphological characteristics. The plants from Swiss seeds were the tallest and also started to develop flowers after about 3½ months. The plants grown from Lebanese and South African seeds had not reached the stage of flowering before being harvested.

In connection with the micromorphological aspects it should be emphasized that the large glandular hairs that are so characteristic of "commercial" marihuana and of hashish were found *only in the flowering tops of the plants originating from the Swiss seeds:* and even there they were very rare. These glands are therefore closely connected with the flowering and fruiting tops of the plants, and it might therefore seem that they are responsible for the production of the cannabis resin found in those parts of the plants that make up the narcotic drug. It therefore came as a surprise to note that *both the flowering and the non-flowering plants from the three localities gave a strongly positive Beam test result* (a violet colour with a 5% KOH solution in ethanol), which should indicate the presence of *cannabidiol* and *cannabidiolic acid,* implying that these are produced in all green parts of the plant.

I would like to point out that as the chemical study of our material has barely begun, I am unable at this moment to say more about the chemical aspects.

References

Farmilo and Charles, G., A Review of Some Recent Results on the Chemical Analysis of Cannabis. ST/SOA-SER.S/4. Geneva U.N. Secretariat (1961).

Korte, F. and Sieper, H., Recent Results of Hashish Analysis. In *Hashish: Its Chemistry and Pharmacology,* p. 15. Ciba Foundation Study Group. No. 21. London 1965.

Thoms, H. and Brandt, W., *Handbuch der praktischen und wissenschaftlichen Pharmazie,* Bd. V. Berlin—Wien 1929.

Wallis, T. E., *Textbook of Pharmacognosy.* 5. Ed. London 1967.

DISCUSSION 1: BOTANICAL ASPECTS

(a) Chemovars and Cultivars

Mechoulam We know from the literature, from our own work and from others' here, that there are considerable chemotaxonomic differences in the different races, the "varieties" as we have been used to calling them until now. One finds plants in which there is cannabidiolic acid and apparently not tetrahydrocannabinolic acid, the precursor of tetrahydrocannabinol. Today we know about 50 typical components of cannabis.

We have recently found other differences in the THC acids themselves, of which I shall say more later. For the moment, calling one "A" and another "B", we have not been able to find both A and B in the same hashish samples: we find either one, or the other. So probably there is a chemotaxonomic difference.

Schultes Was the hashish in your experiments known to be collected from one field at one time, or was it collected a month apart, or from different fields? Was your piece of hashish large enough to have been of heterogeneous origin, or did you control its source?

Mechoulam Hashish in the Middle East comes from Lebanon, and it is big business there, so I tend to assume that the pieces come from one field. The women there make "soles" of hashish—they can collect enough from one field—and then we get them from the police. We know that the soles that we found did not contain both A and B. The ones that contained B did not contain A. We have not looked at many soles yet, just a few.

Shulgin Is there a possibility that the Acid B, the new cannabinolic acid, might arise as an artifact from an abnormal condensation from the cannabidiolic acid?

Mechoulam Cannabidiolic acid B is the thermodynamically less stable of the two acids. Given a chance, it converts into the A acid, so if anything the other one is formed first. But again, we have not done the experiments because they have to be done on the plant. We have no evidence that A is formed from B. In the laboratory we can do that, and I see no reason why the plant should not do it directly.

Agurell Some hashish smokers of Stockholm enclose it in a little tinfoil, which they heat over a couple of lighted matches. I don't think this would cyclize the cannabidiol; but anyway, they know you get a better quality if you heat the preparation first.

Joyce Some British cannabis smokers also heat it with matches, and others have been known to bury it, presumably getting a little spontaneous combustion this way. They claim that this increases the yield.

Fairbairn   Dr. Schultes, are you satisfied with the evidence that there are two chemical races—or do you feel that plants at different stages of development show these differences?

Schultes   I think we could say that there are chemovars. But there is also evidence that they may have different chemical constituents at different times of their growth. These may change, and not be the same chemovar in another area, another climate, another environment. This is not unknown; it is very common, for example, in some of the Solanaceous plants that are grown for atropine production: you cannot grow them in certain places. The digitalis plant was introduced in 1870 to Colombia; it does well in the Andes. A pharmacologist who wanted to start an industry in South America brought the best race from Switzerland, a roughly comparable situation, to the Andes. They have never yet found the glycoside in any of the plants grown in the Northern Andes. So I think the chemovar is something which cannot easily be defined. Dr. Stearn might have something further to say about this.

Stearn   We know now in the history of cultivated plants, even lettuces, that you get indefinable differentiations that affect the way they grow. This is probably true with a number of species. I have helped to introduce digitalis into various places, and you do not get the same results when you grow them in different places; this may very well be true of cannabis. The yield of cannabis in this country is said to vary according to the summer that we have. With very hot summers, there are far more resin glands on cannabis grown at Kew than at other times.

Fairbairn   What you say is quite true in our own experience. We also grow cannabis under artificial illumination and ultraviolet light, and even with the same cultivar we are getting environmental effects.

Paton   Would you expect breeding for oil to be associated with resin or not?

Schultes   I would not think so, but one might influence the other if you bred for one of them, selectively.

Crombie   If some of them produce known narcotic principles, what is the genetic relationship here? One would imagine that there was a genetic difference.

Schultes   Not necessarily. It is not true in the case of alkaloidal plants.

Halbach   If there is a lesson to be learned from what we have heard from Dr. Schultes—that there are no species, but at best varieties, of cannabis—then it ought to have been applied more than ten years ago to the attempts of the German botanists to breed a cannabis devoid of narcotic properties or even devoid of resin. There was a great hope at that time, that one might be able to authorise plantation of this

particular—what was called "species"—in order to do away with the
narcotic dangers. Of course, it was realised immediately that this
species would in any case form hybrids with what was already there
and that the wild species could not be uprooted. The idea was therefore really given up, but it would have been easier still if one had been
able to conclude firmly that there are no different species. It is worth
making the point in order to prevent people from going astray again.
Schultes   Possibly at that time the botanists and the chemists never
sat down together; this is a relatively recent approach. This problem
still exists, because botanists give a very definite meaning to species,
variety, family, order and so forth, and these words are loosely used
by non-botanists and even by agricultural specialists. It is not so much a
problem with chemists and pharmacologists, but it is a tremendous problem in the law courts. Lawyers have based whole cases on the fact
that their client did not possess *Cannabis indica,* but *Cannabis sativa.*
Mechoulam   Dr. Schultes has reported (Schultes, R. E. 1967 in:
"Ethnopharmacologic Search for Psychoactive Drugs" ed. Efron, D. H.
et al. p. 302. Washington D.C. Department of Health, Education and
Welfare) that the tree *Olmedioperebea sclerophylla* (fam. *Moraceae*)
is used by the natives in the Amazon river area as a psychotomimetic
snuff: "rapé dos indios"). Very few, if any, other plants, of the same
family are used as hallucinogens. *Cannabis sativa* was once considered
a member of the *Moraceae* family. It should be of interest to identify
the active principles of *Olmedioperebea.* They may be related to the
cannabinoids.
Schultes   This plant is a tremendous jungle tree with very fleshy
fruits that do not last long, as monkeys and birds quickly eat them.
Study of their active principles has not yet yielded a substance with
psychotomimetic effects.
Mechoulam   A typical expression of the strain differences in *Cannabis*
itself may be found by a chemotaxonomic investigation of the numerous cannabinoids. It is well known that cannabis resin of different
origin varies in its chemical content enormously. For critical chemotaxonomic work fresh plants would have to be used.

(b) Determination of Geographical Origins
Stearn   There are also gross differences in the resins from different
sources. One type of resin from Pakistan is stamped with the makers'
name and of a very dark brown colour; resins from elsewhere have
lighter colours, and so on. The police say that there are also variations
in the rough tops and in the colour, that they can roughly pin down
geographically. Is this so?

Braenden   The determination of the geographic origin of cannabis
is a very complex problem differing in many ways from that of the
determination of the origin of opium. For opium, authenticated samples are available from most of the regions where opium is produced.
In the case of cannabis it would be extremely difficult to have an
adequate range of authenticated samples since most is derived from
unauthorized cultivation. Opium is also a very stable product, unlike
cannabis, in which considerable changes may occur even after relatively short periods of storage. Certain differences in the appearance
of samples of hashish are mainly due to variations in the methods of
collection. For example, in some regions the resin is collected by
threshing and subsequently pressed into cakes or plates; in other
regions, the resin adheres to the rubber aprons of the collectors as
they walk through the fields and is afterwards scraped off.
Razdan   In Tibet it is believed that a greater yield is obtained when
the collectors walk naked through the fields so that the resin adheres
to their bodies.
Mechoulam   All the typical compounds are perhaps from females,
and females are known to give the black compounds, and many-
coloured compounds, just on staying around. We have found that
samples of hashish start going black as do even the pure synthetic
compounds if they are exposed for some time to the air.
      There is a suggestion that the origin may eventually be identified
by neutron-activation analysis. Samples from many parts are needed
as well as an atomic reactor. It has been done and we have somebody
who is willing to do it on identified specimens.
A. S. Curry   We also use neutron-activation analysis, though arc
emission may prove to be a simpler and quicker method of identifying
trace elements. The subject of trace elements in cannabis is a big one.
Professor Webb at the School of Mines has prepared a 28 trace element
map at one square mile intervals for the whole of England, Wales and
Northern Ireland. This map reminds me very much indeed of Dr. Haney's
distribution patterns in Illinois. Trace metals may also influence
cannabis production: this may be related to the enzymatic differences
in plants that are responsible for the A and B acids.
Scigliano   Using the term "the geographic source" to refer to the
seed rather than the product, we have generally found that you cannot distinguish one plant from the other. Plants from a Turkish seed,
two fibre-producing seeds from a French source, two seeds from Italy,
and a seed from Sweden cannot be distinguished one from the other.
      With regard to colour, much can sometimes be attributed to the
clay or the soil that suppliers of low integrity mix in as a diluent;

with some samples when the hashish is dissolved out there is a lot of mud left at the bottom of the test tube.

Lister Is there any relationship between the duration of light-dark cycles to which the plants are exposed and their rate of growth or the formation of any of the active constituents?

Haney We have found that this influences the sex ratio, so it may also perhaps influence the amount of active substances.

(c) Sex

Shulgin I am struck by the fact that some rather simple chemical, such as carbon monoxide, can actually affect the sex distribution. Which sex carries the sex-information in the cannabis, and for how long a period can this meiotic sensitivity be influenced chemically?

Haney I am not sure if any information is available in reply to your first question. On your second question, this is carried for some length of time. Very young plants approximately only one to two weeks old were modified as a result of only one to two days exposure, at a time when they were obviously nowhere near sexual maturity. Carbon monoxide is a rather reactive compound.

Miras Under bad conditions the plant may be monoecious. It still produces a little resin, mostly containing cannabinolic acids, but also tetrahydrocannabinol.

Haney Harrison found that the beginning of the change from male to female produced by carbon monoxide was first indicated by her-maphroditic flowers, in which the organs of both sexes were present in the same flower as well as in the same plant. The latter does occur, but the U.S. Department of Agriculture experts report thay they have never seen a monoecious plant in the hundreds of specimens that they have examined from police sources.

Scigliano We have grown a monoecious plant in which the female blossom is on the upper part of the plant, whereas the male flower is on the lower portion.

Crombie Can one sex a seed?

Haney I do not think anyone has tried to do so.

Kusevic Is there a general tendency for world cultivation of cannabis to increase or decrease owing to the production of synthetic fibres? Can these replace cannabis?

Schultes Hemp fibre production in the United States has gone down mainly because of the cost of labour; it is cheaper to buy fibres from abroad. I doubt if synthetic fibres are substituting for hemp fibre to any great extent. Although there are now synthetic fibres for clothing, more cotton is being produced in the world than ever before. Whether this is true or not of cannabis I do not know.

Joyce   Approximately how many counties are there in the United
States? i.e., what is the asymptote to which Dr. Haney's exponential
curve is tending? What does it mean if a sample has not been collected
from a particular area? How comparable are the various collection
techniques, and what is the significance of the absence of a figure?
i.e., what is known about the missing denominator?
Haney   I am not sure. We certainly cannot take these data to be hard
and fast because of the variability in collecting methods and the
variability of the measurements made upon the collections.
I would guess there may be 2,400-3,000 counties in the United
States, and we have now had specimens from 800 or so of them, i.e.
about one in three.

(d) Biosynthesis

Fairbairn   Loomis tried to incorporate laevulonic acid into the
volatile oil glands of certain plants and just could not get it in,
although it is a precursor of these terpenes; he could get carbon
dioxide in, and it may be that there is a barrier which prevents the
precursor passing into these glandular trichomes.
Mechoulam   Surprisingly, nobody has yet proved that laevulonic
acid is a precursor for monoterpenes. It is obvious, and everybody
says so, but many very good people have tried to show it and have
failed.
Korte   Two years ago we injected C_{14} laevulonic acid into the growing
plant and isolated some tetrahydrocannabinol from the radioactive
part of the root, but the conversion rate is less than five per cent or so.
Shulgin   I would like to return to the most important question:
whether THC, presumed to be the active material in marihuana, is or
is not present in the native parent plant. Dr. Korte was not able to
find it there, yet Dr. Miras has reported a radiographic spot from
fresh plants that corresponds to it.
Miras   You can also find THC in small amounts in fresh seeds.
Shulgin   Was THC present, as such, in Dr. Agurell's thin layer chro-
matography, of extracts from fresh plants?
Agurell   No. We had cannabidiolic acid as a 95-97% constituent but
no more than traces, if that, of THC.
Haney   Were the plants you were working with grown outdoors, or
under glass?
Miras   Outdoors.
Agurell   In a greenhouse, with u.v. tubing.
Haney   Ultra-violet light is a very important factor.
Mechoulam   We do not believe that ultraviolet light makes a difference.

We have tried irradiating pure samples of cannabidiolic acid and THC acid with sensitizers. We get many reactions but decarboxylation does not seem to be one of these. So *if* natural and laboratory irradiation are comparable, there is no decarboxylation.

(e) Forensic Identification of Cannabis

Fairbairn We place a great deal of reliance for purposes of identification on the glandular trichomes; is there any likelihood of confusion with any other plant having similar trichomes in your experience?

Nordal Not as far as I know.

Joyce It is said from time to time that hashish from certain areas has been mixed with stramonium or with opium-like substances, and so on. What difference does this make to the identification?

Nordal The solanaceous plants like *Datura, Belladonna* and so on have very characteristic anatomical elements, so they can easily be found in pipes when mixed with cannabis. Microscopic detection of opium is very difficult, but chemical methods for the alkaloids, as for those of the solanaceous plants, are available.

Joyce To what extent would the microscopical appearance of the residues be changed by smoking them in cigarettes rather than in a pipe? More of our users smoke cannabis in cigarettes than pipes.

Nordal If uncombusted or semi-combusted remnants of the whole material are left in the ends of the cigarettes you can use the same methods as for pipes. If the hashish is put in the middle of the cigarette, or if only the filter remains, you can extract the unsmoked tip chemically.

A. S. Curry The Dangerous Drugs Act in this country defines cannabis as the "flowering tops" of any species of the genus Cannabis. How do you prove it is the flowering tops? Do you look for pollen, or ovular tissue? I notice that in the new Act the sex is not defined.

Fairbairn Glandular hairs, the presence of the active ingredients, show that this must be a flowering plant and another section of the Act says: "Any extract thereof". That is where the resin comes in. In the vast majority of samples, it is very rare not to have seeds.

Stearn The scanning electron microscope can also provide evidence for use in court. At higher magnifications than 300x you cannot see so much. The cannabis trichomes have a rather distinctive structure at the bottom that I have not seen in any others.

PART TWO

CHEMISTRY

1 Synthesis of (−)-tetrahydrocannabinol and Analogous Compounds

T. Petrzilka

The chemical investigation of hashish and marihuana began at the beginning of the 19th century, but it was almost 100 years before the first defined compound was isolated in pure form, and it took another 30 years until the main features of this compound, which was called cannabinol, were elucidated by the elegant work of Cahn and his group (see Mechoulam, Braun and Gaoni, 1967).

Our own synthetic work originally used as a starting point a proposal made by my friend and colleague Professor Eschenmoser. It was thought that the cannabidiol molecule could be bisected into olivetol and cyclic terpene parts:

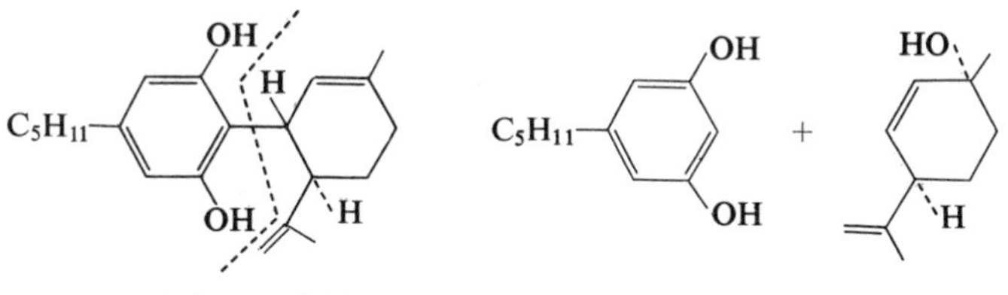

(−)-trans-CBD   (+)-cis-Menthadienol

If it were possible to combine olivetol with (+)-cis-menthadienol to give an ether, it should be possible by means of a Claisen-rearrangement to form the desired trans-cannabidiol under stereochemically controlled conditions. It was hoped that ether formation could be brought about by means of N,N-dimethylformamide-dineopentyl-acetal, which had proved to be a very useful re-agent for the esterification of carboxylic acids.

79

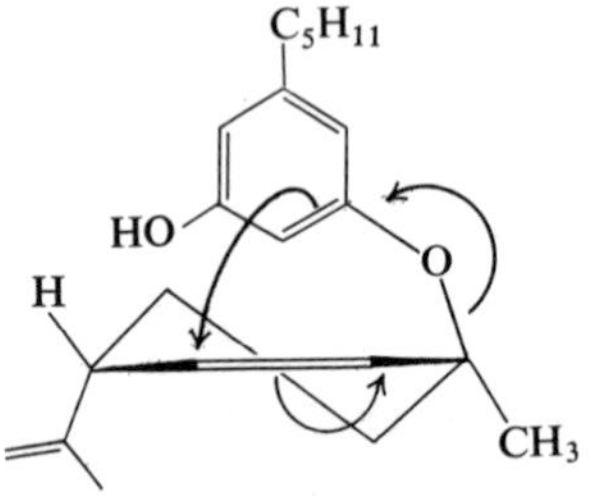

cis-Menthadienyl-Ether 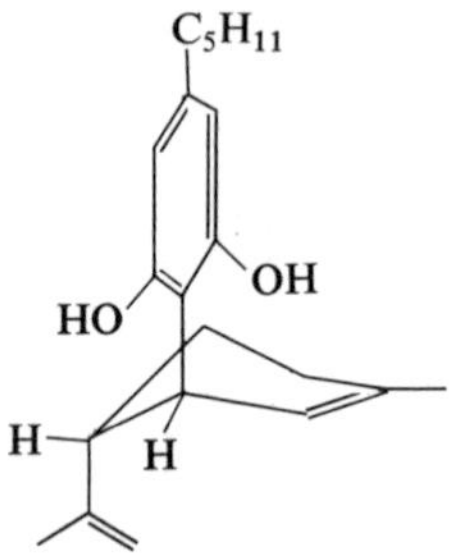   trans-CBD

When we tried this reaction at room temperature three products were obtained, namely (−)-cannabidiol in 25% yield, 4-menthadienyl-olivetol in 35% yield, and 2,4-dimenthadienyl-olivetol in 5% yield:

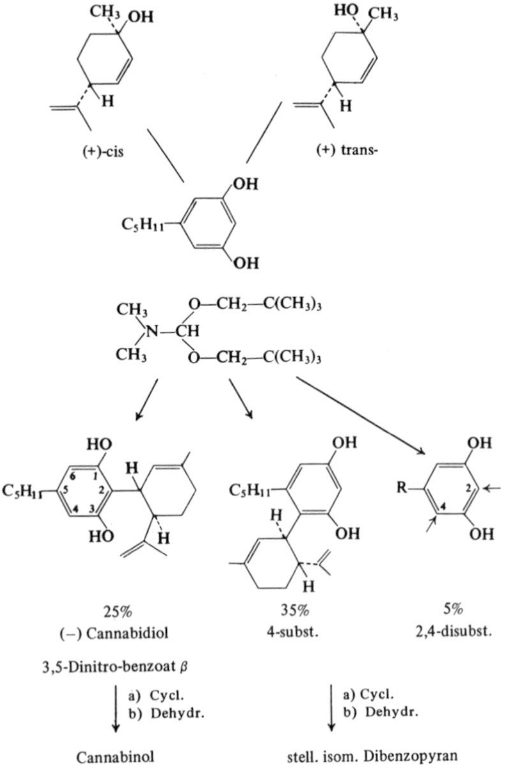

| 25% | 35% | 5% |
| (−) Cannabidiol | 4-subst. | 2,4-disubst. |

3,5-Dinitro-benzoat β

a) Cycl.
b) Dehydr.

Cannabinol

a) Cycl.
b) Dehydr.

stell. isom. Dibenzopyran

Since (−)-cannabidiol was formed under conditions (room temperature)
where usually no Claisen-rearrangement occurs, and since the reaction
of (+)-trans-menthadienol under the same conditions gave the same
reaction products in essentially the same yields, whereas under the
proposed Claisen-rearrangement mechanism it should have yielded
the *cis*-fused cannabidiol, we were led to propose a different reaction
mechanism:

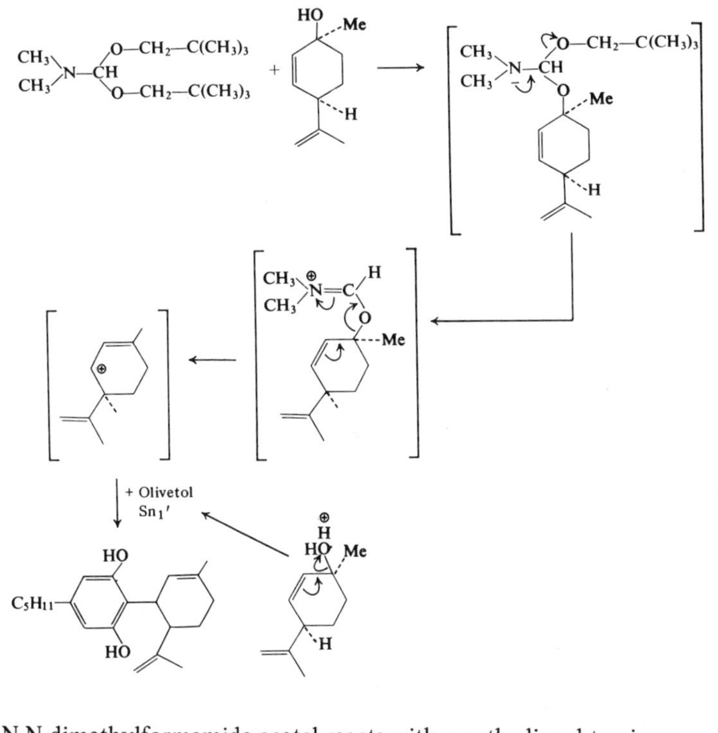

N,N-dimethylformamide-acetal reacts with menthadienol to give a
mixed acetal; after protonation this could eliminate neo-pentylalcohol,
leading to an immonium-ion, which possesses an excellent leaving
group in the dimethylformamide-part of the molecule. On elimination
of dimethylformamide, a carbonium ion would be formed; this could
then react with olivetol in the sense of a nucleophilic substitution
reaction.

Further support for this reaction mechanism was found in the fact

TABLE 1. *Condensation under the influence of weak acids*

Catalyst	Yield (%)	
	(−)-2 substituted Olivetol	(−)-4 substituted Olivetol
N,N-Dimethylformamide dineopentylacetal	21	32
Oxalic acid dihydrate	23.5	34.5
Zinc chloride anhydrous	17	38
2-Hydroxypyridine	15	20.5
2-Hydroxy-5-nitropyridine	7	19
Picric acid	19	20
Maleic acid	21.5	32

that condensation between olivetol and menthadienol could also be brought about by weak acids. As can be seen from Table 1, a number of weak to medium strong acids yielded the same products in about the same yields.

When our new condensation reaction with N,N-dimethylformamide dineopentyl acetal was applied to 4-carbethoxy-olivetol, for which Korte described a synthesis in 1960, 4-carbethoxy-cannabidiol could be isolated in a yield of 42%. On hydrolysis with sodium hydroxide solution, (−)-cannabidiol which was identical in all respects with the natural product from cannabis resulted:

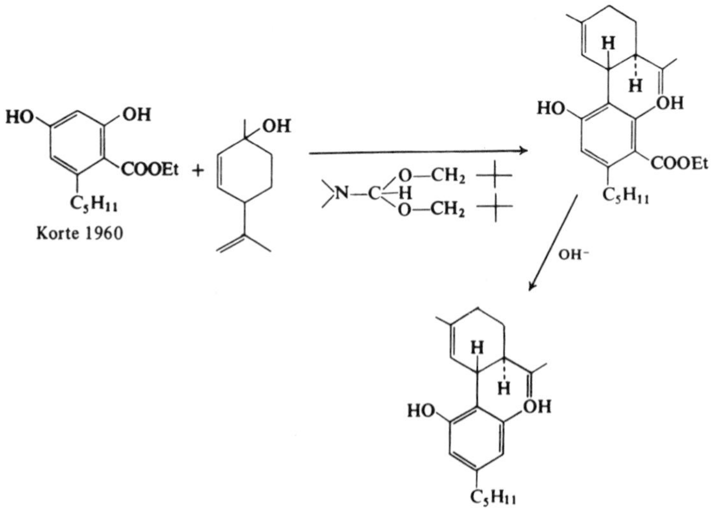

TABLE 2. *Condensation under the influence of strong acids*

Catalyst	Yield %		
	$(-)-\Delta^8$-THC	$(-)-\Delta^9$-THC	$(-)$-1-n Amyl-3-hydroxy-Δ^8-6a, 10a-trans-tetra-hydro-dibenzo (b d) pyran
Toluene-p-sulphonic acid	53	–	13
0.05% Hydrogen chloride in tert.-butyl alcohol	13	–	25
Trifluoroacetic acid	55	–	13
0.0005 N Ethanolic hydrochloric acid	2.3	1	little

When strong acids were used as catalysts for the condensation reaction, again, 3 reaction-products were obtained (Table 2). These were $(-)-\Delta^8$-THC in 53% yield, identical in all respects with the authentic product, isolated from hashish by Hoffman, Hively and Mosher (see Mechoulam *et al.*, 1967), 4-substituted, cyclised olivetol in 13% and a 2,4 disubstituted cyclised olivetol in about 5% yield:

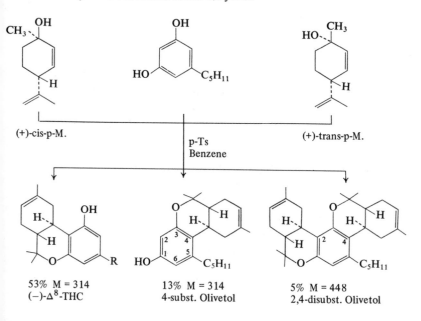

(+)-cis-p-M.   p-Ts Benzene   (+)-trans-p-M.

53% M = 314
$(-)-\Delta^8$-THC

13% M = 314
4-subst. Olivetol

5% M = 448
2,4-disubst. Olivetol

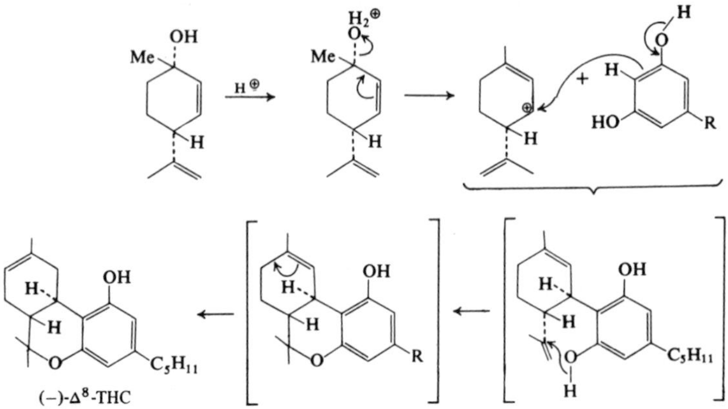

(−)-Δ^8-THC
Stable

(−)-Δ^9-THC
Unstable

So according to our reaction scheme the carbonium ion had formed first, then nucleophilic substitution had taken place, and after that ring closure had occurred under the influence of strong acid, and finally the double bond had shifted to the more stable Δ^8-position (see above).

This shift of the double bond was undesirable, since the natural active principle of cannabis has the double bond in the Δ^9-position. We therefore sought conditions which would bring about condensation and ring-closure, but avoid shifting the double bond. However, with the exception of one experiment, in which a small amount of Δ^9-THC could be isolated, no such conditions could be formed.

Since (+)-p-menthadienol is made from (+)-limonene, which itself has been connected with the system of d(+)-glyceraldehyde, our synthesis of (−)-cannabidiol and (−)-tetrahydrocannabinol represents a proof of the absolute configuration of these compounds, which had not previously been known with certainty.

As early as 1940, Adams (see Mechoulam et al., 1967) had tried to prove the chirality of (−)-cannabidiol by converting it to a tetrahydro-compound, which on oxidation with $KMnO_4$ yielded a menthane-carboxylic acid; this same acid could be synthesized by converting (−)-menthol to menthyl-chloride which on treatment with Mg and CO_2 gave the carboxylic acid. The two acids in the form of their amides gave no depression of the melting point and therefore were

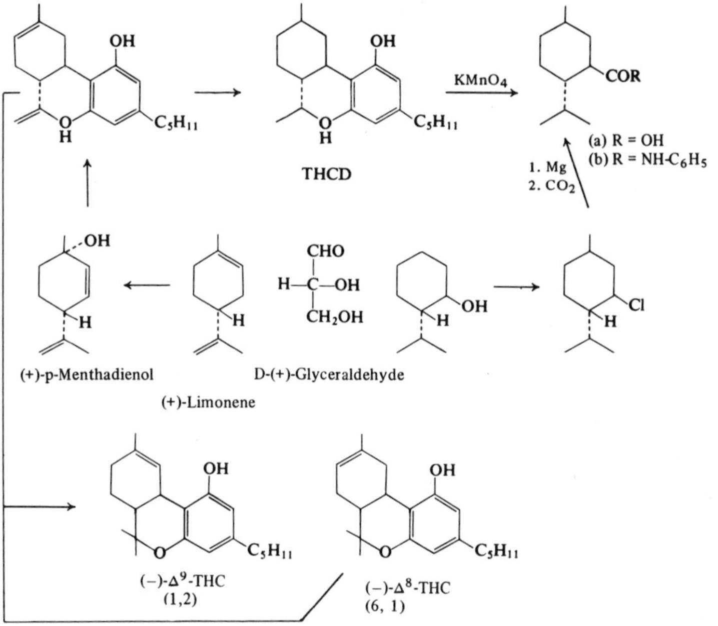

THCD

(a) R = OH
(b) R = NH-C₆H₅

1. Mg
2. CO₂

(+)-p-Menthadienol

D-(+)-Glyceraldehyde

(+)-Limonene

CHO
H—C—OH
CH₂OH

(−)-Δ⁹-THC
(1,2)

(−)-Δ⁸-THC
(6, 1)

thought to be identical. However, since no optical rotations of those compounds were measured, the proof was not valid. In 1967 Mechoulam repeated Adams' work (Mechoulam *et al.*, 1967) this time measuring optical rotations, and it was gratifying to see that his results agreed with ours.

We used our new method for preparing a number of homologues, in much the same way as Adams had done in the 1940's; however, our new compounds have the stereo-chemistry and position of the double bond as in the natural products from cannabis (Table 3). For the preparation of most of these we were able to use the procedures given by Adams, with the exception of α,α-dimethyl-THC. Whereas Adams used ether as a solvent in the methylation reaction of the nitrile, we found that under these conditions only the monomethyl-derivative was formed; when the reaction was run in dimethoxyethane or DMF the dimethyl compound was formed in good yield. Furthermore, we found that under the conditions used for the elimination of the keto function (reduction to the alcohol, elimination of the elements of water according to the method of Tschugaeff), rearrangements of the side chain occurred. This difficulty could be avoided by

TABLE 3. *Homologues of (−)-Δ⁸-3,4-trans-THC*

Starting material R =	Yield (%)	
	Substitution at 2	Substitution at 4
−H, Resorcinol	15.9	32.2
−CH₃, Orcinol	45.5	27.3
−C₅H₁₁, Olivetol	52.8	13.3
−CH−C₄H₉ 　| 　CH₃	71.6	5.0
−CH—CH−C₅H₁₁ 　|　　| 　CH₃　CH₃	61.4	8.6
CH₃ 　| −C—C₄H₉ 　| 　CH₃	93.2	2.8

$$
\begin{array}{c}
\downarrow \\
\text{HO}\overset{2}{\diagdown}\diagup\text{OH} \\
\diagup\underset{4}{\diagdown} \\
\text{R}
\end{array}
$$

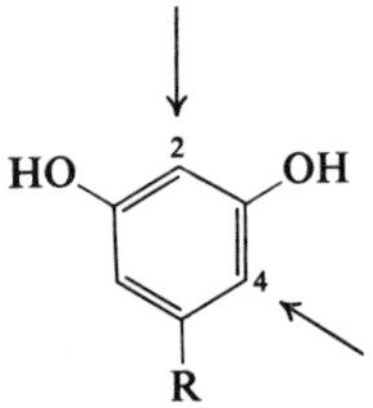

forming the thioketal of the ketone and reduction of the latter to the hydrocarbon:

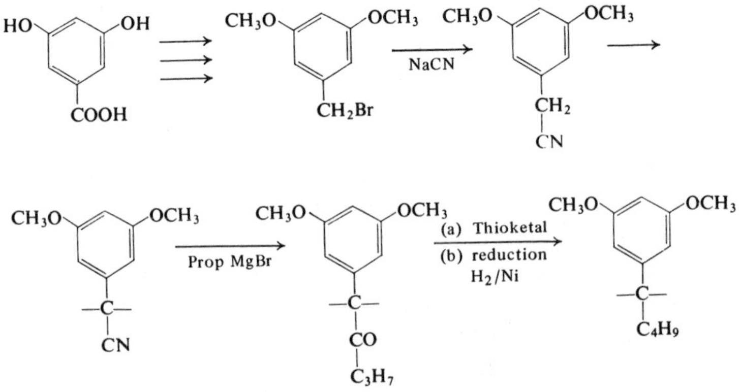

$$
\begin{array}{ccccc}
\text{HO} & \text{OH} & & \text{CH}_3\text{O} & \text{OCH}_3 \\
& & \Longrightarrow & & \\
& & \Longrightarrow & & \xrightarrow{\text{NaCN}} \\
& & \Longrightarrow & & \\
\text{COOH} & & & \text{CH}_2\text{Br} &
\end{array}
$$

$$
\begin{array}{c}
\text{CH}_3\text{O} \quad\quad \text{OCH}_3 \\
\text{CH}_2 \\
\text{CN}
\end{array} \longrightarrow
$$

$$
\begin{array}{c}
\text{CH}_3\text{O} \quad \text{OCH}_3 \\
-\text{C}- \\
\text{CN}
\end{array}
\xrightarrow{\text{Prop MgBr}}
\begin{array}{c}
\text{CH}_3\text{O} \quad \text{OCH}_3 \\
-\text{C}- \\
\text{CO} \\
\text{C}_3\text{H}_7
\end{array}
\xrightarrow[\substack{\text{(b) reduction} \\ \text{H}_2/\text{Ni}}]{\text{(a) Thioketal}}
\begin{array}{c}
\text{CH}_3\text{O} \quad \text{OCH}_3 \\
-\text{C}- \\
\text{C}_4\text{H}_9
\end{array}
$$

It should be noted that the bulkier the alkyl side chain the more the substitution takes place in the 2-position, and the smaller it is, the

more the menthyl-residue enters the 4-position. This is probably due
to steric hindrance of the neighbouring positions to R.

Since we had found a convenient one-step synthesis of Δ^8-THC,
which has the double bond in the more stable position, we were faced
with the problem of shifting the double bond to the less stable Δ^9 position.
Such a method had been described by Kierstead and others at the
Hoffman—La Roche Company. 9-Hydroxy-hexahydrocannabinol had
been treated with Lucas-reagent to give 9-chlorohexahydrocannabinol
in 55% yield. This upon treatment with sodium hydride in THF gave
a mixture of 74% Δ^9- and 26% Δ^8-THC. From this mixture the desired
Δ^9-isomer could be isolated in 15% yield via the crystalline m- nitro-
toluenesulphonate derivative. So, although conversion to the desired
Δ^9 compound had been achieved in a relatively good yield, the isolation of the pure Δ^9-isomer from the mixture proved to be a tedious
process. What was desired was a method for a quantitative conversion
to the Δ^9-isomer, which would make separation and purification
unnecessary.

When we treated Δ^8-THC with hydrochloric acid in methylene
chloride solution in the presence of $ZnCl_2$, a quantitative yield of the
9-chloro-compound was obtained. When the chloro-compound was
run into an excess of potassium-t-amylate in benzene, elimination of
the elements of hydrochloric acid took place with quantitative formation of the desired Δ^9-isomer. The compound proved to be identical
in all respects (IR, NMR, Rf, optical rotation, etc.) with the active
principle from cannabis:

(±)-Δ^8-THC   (−)-9-Chloro-HHC

(−)-9-Chloro-HHC-anion   100%
                                 (−)-Δ^9-THC

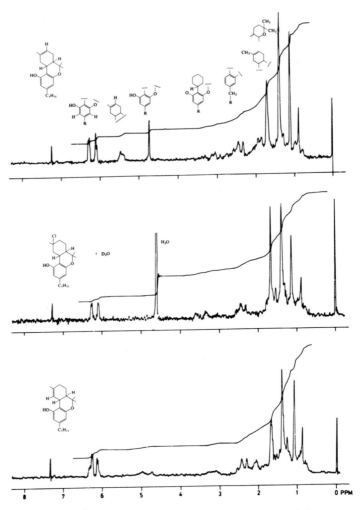

Fig. 1. NMR spectra showing addition and elimination of the
elements of hydrochloric acid with Δ8-THC.

We assume that with the base the phenolate-anion is formed, which
then initiates abstraction of a proton and a chlorine anion. The fact
that the 4-substituted chlorocompound on treatment with potassium-
t-amylate is left unchanged seems to lend support to this view, because
in this case the phenolic anion is too far away from the methylene

group for reaction. Addition and elimination of the elements of hydrochloric acid to Δ^8-THC can be nicely followed by NMR-spectroscopy
(Fig. 1). The Δ^8-compound shows a characteristic peak for the C8
proton at 5.5 ppm, which disappears on addition of hydrochloric
acid. After elimination of hydrochloric acid a new peak appears at
6.3 ppm, whereas no trace of the peak can be seen at 5.5 ppm.

Some time after our synthesis had appeared, a new synthesis of
THC was published by Mechoulam *et al.,* (1967). His synthesis in
many ways resembles our own, in that here too olivetol is condensed
with a cyclic terpene, namely verbenol, to give 2-verbenyl-olivetol,
which could then be rearranged and cyclized to Δ^8-THC:

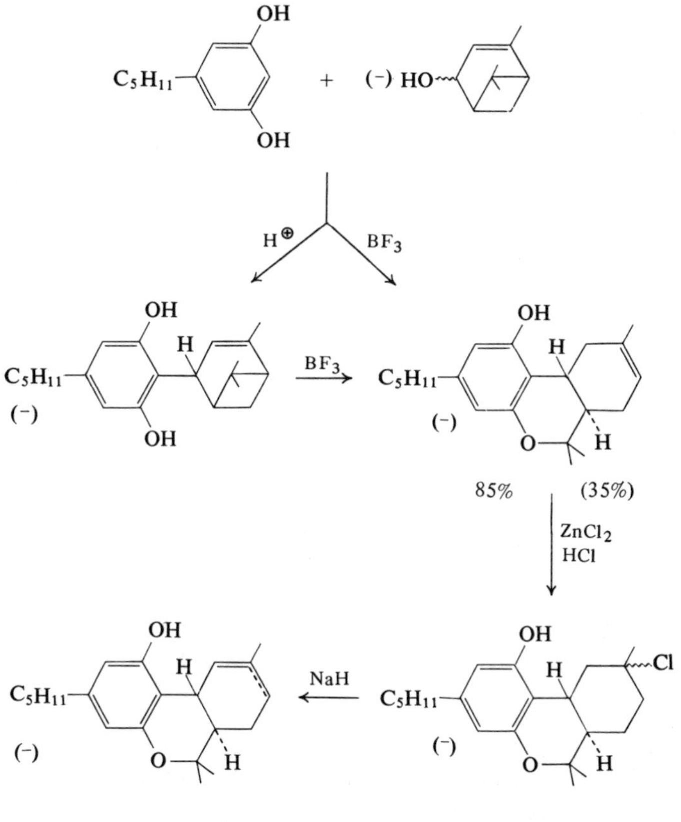

$\Delta^{1,2}$- + $\Delta^{6,1}$-THC

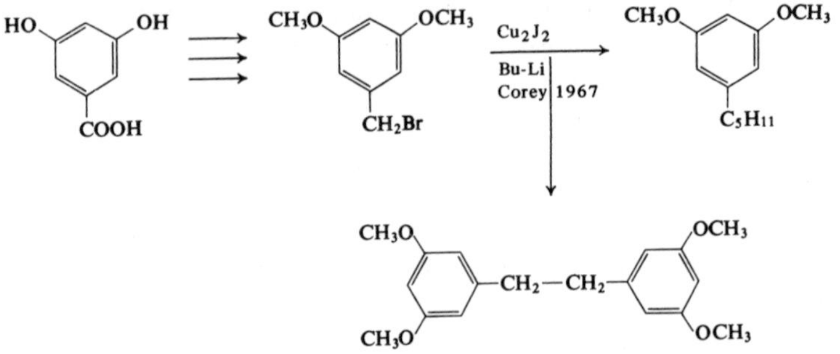

In the course of our synthetic work, we also developed a new synthesis of olivetol, which served us as one of the starting materials. 3,5-dimethoxybenzylbromide can be easily prepared from commercially available resorcinolcarboxylic acid. Reaction of the benzylbromide with butyl lithium and cuprous iodide under the conditions described by Corey and others in 1967 gave a 50% yield of olivetol-dimethylether in one step. No attempt was made to maximise the yields.

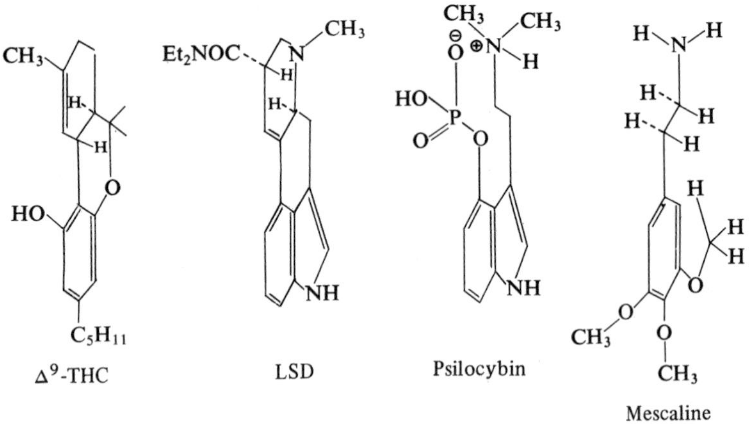

Fig. 2. Δ^9-THC, LSD, Psilocybin, and Mescaline, drawn to demonstrate structural similarities.

In summing up, we may say that we found a practical synthesis for all the main cannabinoids. Moreover, a number of homologues as well as 4-carbethoxy-cannabidiol have been prepared, and finally a new synthesis for olivetol has been described.

In Fig. 2, an attempt is made to correlate structure and hallucino-genic activity of the known hallucinogens. Δ^9-THC, LSD and psilo-cybin all show structural similarities and with some imagination even mescaline can be fitted into this scheme. If one thinks of muscarine, the action of which has been related to its structural resemblance to acetylcholine, one is tempted to think that the hallucinogens may also interfere with some particular enzyme reaction in similar ways.

References

Mechoulam, R., Braun, P. and Gaoni, Y., *J. Amer. Chem. Soc.* 89:4552 (1967).

Mechoulam, R. and Gaoni, Y., *Fortschr. Chem. Org. Naturst.* 25:175 (1967).

Jen, T. Y., Hughes, G. A. and Smith, H., *J. Amer. Chem. Soc.* 89:4551 (1967).

Petrzilka, T., Haefliger, W. and Sikemeier, C., *Helv. Chim. Acta* 52:1102 (1969)

Petrzilka, T., Haefliger, W., Sikemeier, C., Ohloff, G. and Eschenmoser, A., *ibid.* 50:719, (1967).

Petrzilka, T. and Sikemeier, C., *ibid.* 50:1416 (1967).

Petrzilka, T. and Sikemeier, C., *ibid.* 50:2111 (1967).

2 Some Aspects of Cannabinoid Chemistry

R. Mechoulam, A. Shani, B. Yagnitinsky, Z. Ben-Zvi,
P. Braun and Y. Gaoni

The chemistry of hashish constituents (cannabinoid chemistry) has been a very active area of research in the last few years. The newly acquired material makes it impossible, within the time limits of one paper, to survey the whole field or even the advances made since we reviewed the area in 1967 (Mechoulam and Gaoni, 1967). Therefore, I propose to discuss mostly our own work with emphasis on research just completed or still in progress in Jerusalem.

When we started our then very small programme on hashish some 5-6 years ago, our interest in this fascinating field was kindled by the contrast of rich folklore and popular belief with paucity of scientific knowledge. Israel is situated in a part of the world where, for many, hashish is a way of life. Though neither a producer nor a large consumer, Israel is a crossroad for smugglers, mostly Arab bedouin, who get Lebanese hashish from Jordan through the Negev and Sinai deserts to Egypt. Hence the police vaults are full of material waiting for a chemist. There is also no lack of connoisseurs, official or otherwise, who possess an intimate knowledge of Middle Eastern ways and habits as regards this drug. We were told not only of the various psychotomimetic effects caused by hashish but also of its real or imaginary therapeutic value. The drug was said to prolong the sexual act and to have antidepressant and analgesic, especially antimigraine effects.

In contrast, the scientific aspects of the problem were all but neglected. A recent bibliography (U.N. Econ. Social Council, 1965) listed 1860 titles of works bearing partly or entirely on the subject. However, perusal of the literature revealed that in spite of the considerable progress made in the early forties by the groups of Adams and Todd, the main objectives, from the point of view of the natural products chemist had not been achieved. Thus, the active constituent had not been isolated in pure form, its structure was not fully established and hence it had not been synthesized; the only natural cannabinoid whose structure was fully known was cannabinol (*1a*), an

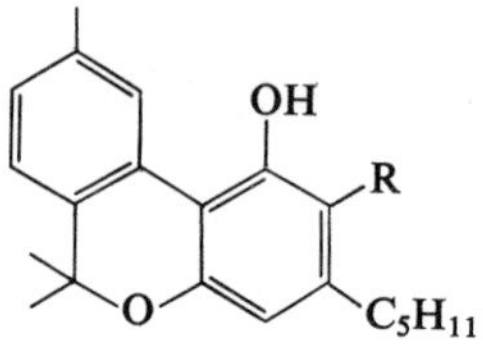

1a. Cannabinol (R = H)
1b. Cannabinolic acid
(R = COOH)

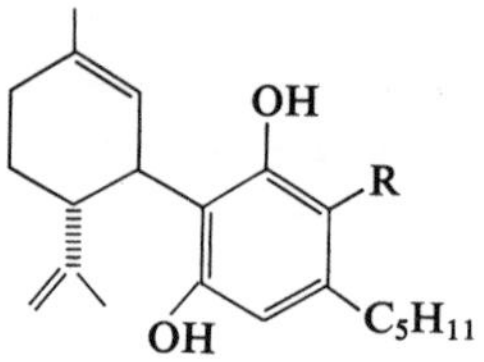

2a. Cannabidiol (R = H)
2b. Cannabidiolic acid
(R = COOH)

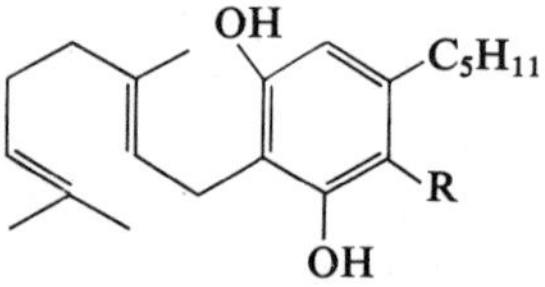

3a. Cannabigerol (R = H)
3b. Cannabigerolic acid
(R = COOH)

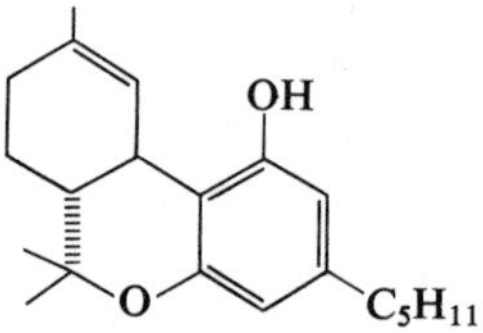

4. Δ^1-Tetrahydrocannabinol
(Δ^1 THC)

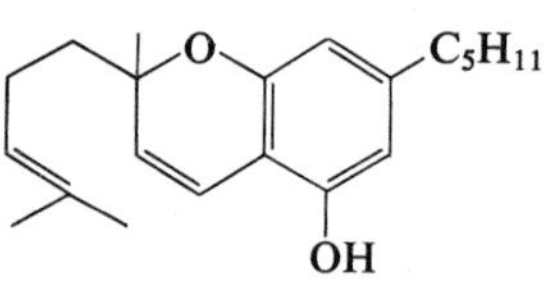

5. Cannabichromene

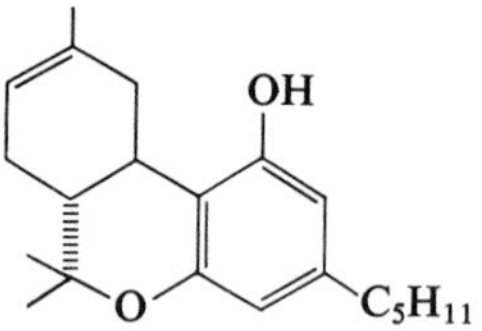

6. $\Delta^{1(6)}$-Tetrahydrocannabinol
($\Delta^{1(6)}$ THC)

Scheme 1.

inactive constituent. This rather surprising lack of chemical knowledge had prevented modern investigations of the biological and clinical aspects. One could not expect biochemists, pharmacologists or clinicians to do serious work with crude plant extracts, whose contents were known to vary widely. Biological results are expected nowadays to be quantitative and reproducible.

Our first foray in the cannabinoid field was a reinvestigation of the separation methods. We found that the method of choice was column chromatography monitored by thin layer chromatography (TLC) and vapour phase chromatography (VPC), analytical tools which were not available to the investigators in the early forties. It was possible to isolate numerous new cannabinoids in addition to cannabidiol (*2a*) and cannabidiolic acid (*2b*), two constituents which had been obtained previously, but whose published structures were found to be incorrect. The structures and stereochemistry of these compounds were investigated mainly by the use of physical methods (nuclear magnetic resonance, NMR; infra-red, IR; ultra-violet and mass spectrometer) as well as by chemical correlations. The following constituents were isolated and their structures elucidated: cannabidiol (*2a*), cannabigerol (*3a*), Δ^1-tetrahydrocannabinol (Δ^1-THC) (*4*), cannabichromene (*5*), cannabidiolic acid (*2b*), cannabinolic acid (*1b*), cannabinol (*1a*),and cannabigerolic acid (*3b*) (Mechoulam and Shvo, 1963; Gaoni and Mechoulam, 1964a, b, 1966; Claussen, von Spulak and Korte, 1966; and Mechoulam and Gaoni, 1965) as well as a few additional ones, whose constitution was fully determined only recently (*vide infra*). The structure of a few components is still being investigated.

The only constituent which was psychotomimetically active *per se* proved to be Δ^1-THC (*4*). Ever since Wollner (1942) reported the isolation of a THC from red oil, it was accepted that compounds of this general type were the active components of marihuana. However, it is doubtful whether a natural THC had ever been isolated in pure form until 1964, when we obtained (Gaoni and Mechoulam, 1964b) for the first time a crystalline derivative, Δ^1-THC dinitrophenylurethane, m.p. 115-6°, which on mild hydrolysis gave Δ^1-THC, pure by VPC and TLC standards. With pure material in hand it was easy to establish its structure by NMR analysis and by correlation with cannabinol (*1a*). A partial synthesis of Δ^1-THC from cannabidiol was also accomplished.* Δ^1-THC is by far the largest, if not the only, THC component in Lebanese hashish. We have been unable to detect

---

* This first report on the isolation in pure form of the predominant active Cannabis component, the elucidation of its structure and its partial synthesis is not cited in an international symposium on the chemistry and pharmacology of hashish (Wolstenholme and Knight, 1965), which took place half a year after the publication of the paper.

any $\Delta^{1(6)}$-THC (6) in this hashish, though Hively, Mosher and Hoffmann (1966) found that some marihuana samples contain minor amounts of this isomer. Lerner and Zeffert (1968) reported that the ratio of Δ^1-THC to $\Delta^{1(6)}$-THC in fresh marihuana (with an average total THC content of 1.2%) varies from 99.9/0.1 to 98.8/1.2. In a hashish "sole" the inside part was found to contain 8% THC (ratio of Δ^1 to $\Delta^{1(6)}$ isomers 98/2), while on the outside the THC content was 1.9% (ratio of Δ^1 to $\Delta^{1(6)}$ isomers 95.5/4.5). These figures do not necessarily reflect a certain conversion of Δ^1 into $\Delta^{1(6)}$-THC in hashish, but may be due to preferential dehydrogenation of Δ^1-THC into cannabinol. We have shown that on chloranil dehydrogenation this is indeed the case (Mechoulam, Yagnitinsky and Gaoni, 1968).

The biological activity of pure Δ^1-THC (4) was determined by Grunfeld and Edery (1969), who found that i.v. injection of 0.5 mg/kg of Δ^1-THC in dogs caused severe motor disturbances and a stuporous state. Recovery commenced after 1-1½ hours. Rhesus monkeys after i.v. injection of 0.1 mg/kg became drowsy within 10 minutes, then ptosis appeared accompanied by intermittent head-drops, both of which could be abolished by strong noise. At about 15 minutes following the drug, spontaneous motor activity almost ceased, the animals withdrew into the far corner of the observation cage and assumed a typical crouched position in which they remained for 1 to 1½ hours, if left undisturbed. The authors term this posture "thinker position" because the monkeys have usually a tendency to support their head with one hand and have a typical blank gaze. A "taming" effect was also present, which was particularly striking in naturally aggressive animals. These effects continued for about 2 hours after which they gradually wore off. The animals regained normal behaviour within 3 hours.

Δ^1-THC after intraperitoneal but not subcutaneous administration suppressed the gerbil digging activity (at 10 mg/kg), reduced the rat conditioned avoidance response to electric shock (at 2 mg/kg) and induced a cataleptoid reaction in mice, rats and gerbils (Grunfeld and Edery, 1969). Bicher and Mechoulam (1968) reported that Δ^1-THC and $\Delta^{1(6)}$-THC possess analgesic properties in both mice and rabbits.

The activity of Δ^1-THC on human volunteers was considerably different from that observed in animals (unpublished results). The dose employed was 70γ/kg *per os*. The initial effects were felt within

30 minutes. After a wavelike spell of uncontrollable laughter, which lasted for nearly an hour, most of the volunteers slowly withdrew from contact with other members of the group. The general feeling was one of euphoria and "a deep understanding of the meaning of things". Time sense was distorted. A few volunteers reported increased sensitivity to sound, spatial distortion, mental confusion and depersonalization. After nearly six hours the effects disappeared leaving a sense of mild depression. In one case the effects were entirely different. No euphoria was experienced. Instead, about two hours after receiving a 20 mg dose, the volunteer fell into a panicky, nearly psychotic state, and needed help by the attendant psychiatrist.*

Recently, Isbell, Gorodetzky, Jasinski and Claussen (1967) published similar though more detailed and quantitative observations They found that "effects of doses of 120γ/kg orally or 50γ/kg on smoking were recognized by all patients as being similar to those of marihuana". It has been reported (Claussen and Korte, 1968) that about 98% of Δ^1-THC impregnated in a cigarette is destroyed on smoking. Hence only the remaining 2%, which is vapourized, accounts for the activity and the actual effective minimal dose by this route is 1γ/kg. This places Δ^1-THC in the dose range of LSD. However, the data regarding the percentage of Δ^1-THC destroyed on smoking remains to be confirmed.

It has been suggested, on the basis of VPC observations, that Δ^1-THC may be converted on smoking into $\Delta^{1(6)}$-THC (Taylor, Lenard and Shvo, 1967). We have shown that this isomerization is due to the chromatographic column and so VPC data are not relevant to the problem (Gaoni and Mechoulam, 1966). Controlled smoking experiments, taking into account the preferential oxidation of Δ^1-THC into cannabinol (versus the lower reactivity of $\Delta^{1(6)}$-THC) have yet to be reported. Evaluation of published data (Lerner and Zeffert, 1968; Claussen and Korte, 1968) on this basis seems to suggest that any isomerization on smoking is negligible, or nonexistent.

---

* These observations were never published by the psychiatrists in charge of the experiment, though they were described by one of the present authors (R.M.) in lectures on a number of occasions since they were performed in 1966. On the basis of this experiment, however, we reported that the effective human dose was 3-5 mg (Mechoulam and Gaoni, 1967). Weil, Zinberg and Nelson (1968) have recently published controlled experiments on the effects of marihuana smoking on volunteers.

Mechoulam and Gaoni (1967) have reported that Δ^1-THC was present as 0.4% of a hashish sole 10-15 months old. This amount is too low to account for the activity of hashish, as judged by the data given above. Therefore we have re-examined the problem (unpublished data). A sample of crude hashish was extracted with petroleum-ether until the remaining material showed no activity (rhesus monkey). A VPC determination (at 240°; 2% OV-17 on Chromosorb W) of the total extract indicated the presence of about 5% Δ^1-THC. Other samples showed 5-7% total Δ^1-THC. However, we were unable to isolate or show the presence of more than about 4% Δ^1-THC. The rest of the materials appearing as Δ^1-THC on vapour phase chromatography were found to be mostly, if not exclusively, the two Δ^1-THC acids, 7a and 8a, which at the high temperature in the VPC instrument were decarboxylated to Δ^1-THC. The acid 7a has been isolated by Korte, Haag and Claussen (1965), and Yamauchi, Shoyama, Aramaki, Azuma and Nishioka (1967). The isomeric acid 8a (Mechoulam, Ben-Zvi, Yagnitinsky and Shani, 1969), is a highly crystalline material, m.p. 184°, a most unusual characteristic for a cannabinoid. The acid 8a differs from 7a in its IR spectrum. It shows a strong band at 1735 cm^{-1}, which is absent in 7a. There are also significant differences in the fingerprint region. On TLC 8a is much more polar than 7a. In order to differentiate between the two acids we have named 7a "Δ^1-THC acid A" and 8a we have named "Δ^1-THC acid B." The chemical correlations indicated in Fig. 1 corroborate the structure of acid 8a.

The conversion of 8a into $\Delta^{1(6)}$-THC acid A with borontrifluoride represents a hitherto unreported isomerization in the cannabinoid series. The mechanism of this reaction probably involves addition of the borontrifluoride to the etheric oxygen in 8a, opening of the pyran ring, followed by cyclization to the alternative pyran system and double bond migration.

The presence in hashish of two ΔTHC acids, in addition to Δ^1-THC itself, will undoubtedly complicate analytical and biological work on Cannabis. The acids *per se* are not active when administered i.v. to rhesus monkeys, but decarboxylate on heating (and probably on smoking) to yield active Δ^1-THC. A number of basic problems remain. Are the acids active orally? If the answer is positive, is the activity the same as Δ^1-THC or is it quantitatively different due to slow decarboxylation?

A further component on which we recently worked is cannabicyclol. It is a very minor component, and is not active. On column chromatography it is eluted together with cannabidiol from which it can be separated by silver-nitrate—alumina chromatography. On the basis of physical measurements we deduced that cannabicyclol is a tetracyclic cannabinoid, possessing no double bonds in the terpene moiety.

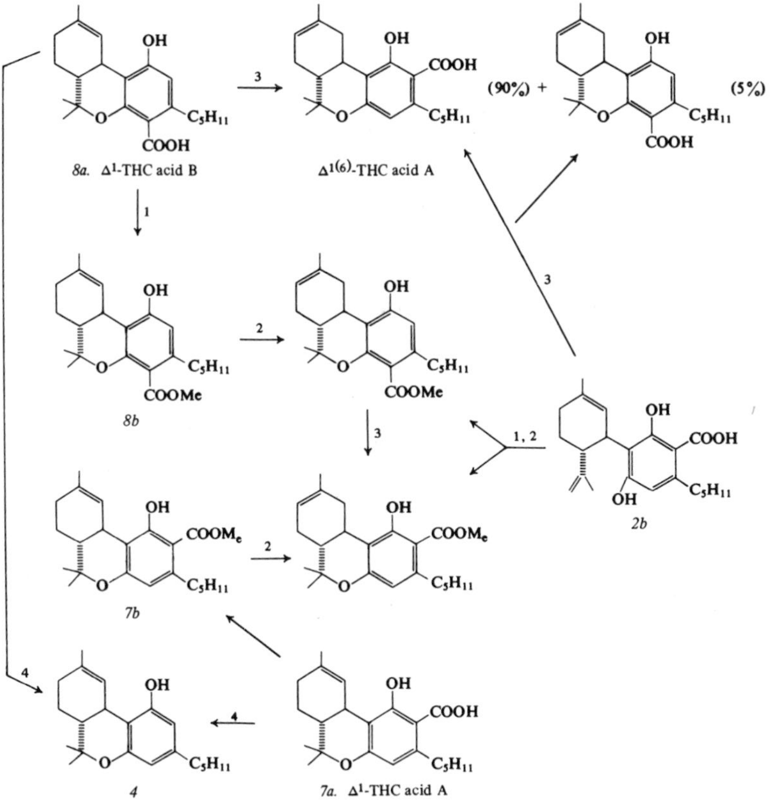

Fig. 1. Interrelations of the THC acids, Reagents: (1) Ch_2N_2; (2) p-toluene sulphonic acid in benzene, 80°; (3) BF_3 etherate, r.t. in CH_2Cl_2; and (4) heat.

We suggested structure 9 as a working hypothesis (Mechoulam and Gaoni, 1967). The same structure was put forward by Claussen, von Spulak and Korte (1968) as a definite representation.

9. Cannabicyclol (old formula)   *10.* Cannabicyclol (new formula)

Scheme 2.

Crombie and Ponsford (1968) re-examined the NMR spectrum of cannabicyclol in a 220 mc instrument. They found that the C_3 proton, which had previously been observed as a broad doublet is in fact a sharp doublet. Hence this proton is adjacent to one proton only. Mainly on the basis of this observation and on NMR decoupling experiments, structure *9* was modified to *10*. This modification has not yet gained general acceptance. Kane and Razdan (1968) consider structure *10* not fully proven and suggest that *9* should not be discarded at the present time. These authors view the NMR and mass spectral data as not satisfactorily explained by structure *10*. They also point out that the thermal conversion (Crombie and Ponsford, 1968) of cannabichromene (*5*) into *10* is hardly acceptable (Woodward-Hoffmann rules). However in a joint communication members of Crombie's group and of our group (Crombie, Ponsford, Shani, Yagnitinsky and Mechoulam, 1968) have shown that the photo-chemical cyclization of *5* into *10* which is in accordance with Woodward-Hoffmann rules, proceeds with ease and in high yields. By contrast the thermal conversion is a low yield one, and is possibly a non-concerted reaction. Cannabicyclol has now been prepared also by an acid treatment of *5* (*vide infra*).

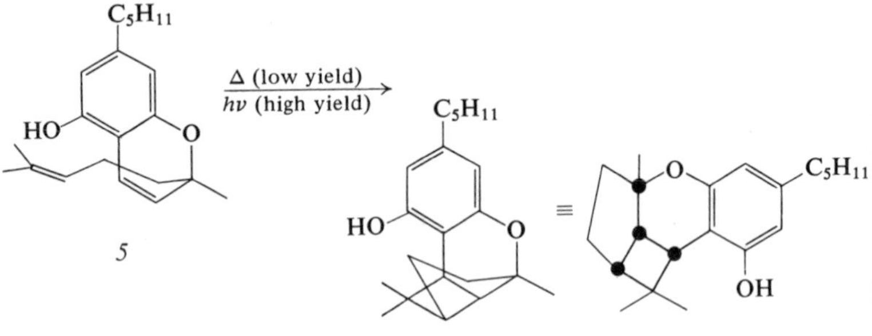

Scheme 3.

Cannabicyclol and cannabichromene from the crude drug, when pure, show no apparent rotation. Cannabichromene could originate as a natural product through asymmetric intermediate or non-stereo-specific (non-enzymic?) processes, and cannabicyclol could form as a result of natural irradiation in the plant, with other constituents acting as sensitizers. On the other hand, it is possible that both compounds are artefacts formed in the crude drug.

Absolute configuration

The absolute configuration at both asymmetric centres C_3 and C_4 in natural Δ^1-THC is (R). This has been established by chemical correlation with (−) menthol (Mechoulam and Gaoni, 1967b) and by syntheses from monoterpenes with known absolute configurations (Mechoulam, Braun and Gaoni, 1967; Petrzilka, Haefliger, Sikemeier, Ohloff and Eschenmoser, 1967).

Syntheses

The isolation and elucidation of the structures of Δ^1-THC and $\Delta^{1(6)}$-THC led to a flurry of synthetic activity. In 1965 we reported the first synthesis of *dl*-cannabidiol and *dl*-Δ^1-THC (Mechoulam and Gaoni, 1966b). It was soon followed by the disclosure of a number of other approaches from academic and industrial laboratories. The easiest synthesis of *dl*-$\Delta^{1(6)}$-THC seems to be the one reported by Taylor, Lenard and Shvo (1967); that of *dl*-Δ^1-THC is a modification of Taylor's experimental procedure developed in our laboratory (unpublished).

Within a few months in 1967, three groups announced successful syntheses of (−) Δ^1-THC (*4*) (Mechoulam, Braun and Gaoni, 1967; Petrzilka and Sikemeier, 1967), (−) $\Delta^{1(6)}$-THC (*6*) (Mechoulam, Braun and Gaoni, 1967; Petrzilka and Sikemeier, 1967; Jen, Hughes and Smith, 1967) and (−) cannabidiol (*2a*) (Petrzilka, Haefliger, Sikemeier, Ohloff and Eschenmoser, 1967). The strategy behind our approach was twofold: (i) the molecules of Δ^1 and $\Delta^{1(6)}$-THC are nearly planar and equally hindered from both sides. Therefore a plausible route to a stereospecific synthesis seemed to us one proceeding via some highly sterically hindered intermediate, which would be attacked from one side only and could later be modified to give not only the natural (3R, 4R) THC derivatives but also the 3S, 4S form.

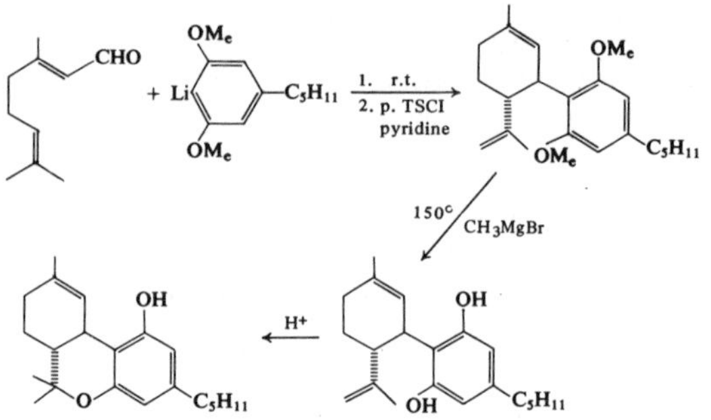

First synthesis of *dl*-cannabidiol and *dl*-Δ^1-THC (Mechoulam and Gaoni, 1966).

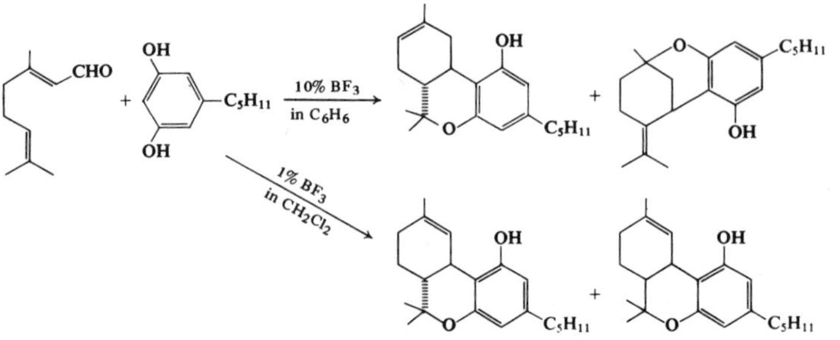

Practical syntheses of *dl*-$\Delta^{1(6)}$ and *dl*-Δ^1-THC.

Scheme 4.

We found that the use of a pinane derivative fulfilled both requirements. In verbenol the bulky dimethyl-methylene bridge provided full stereochemical control of the reactions; all products obtained were 3,4 *trans* exclusively. Also, verbenol was readily available in both the 5(S) and 5(R) forms, to give natural, active (−) $\Delta^{1(6)}$-THC and inactive (+) $\Delta^{1(6)}$-THC.

From a practical viewpoint for the preparation of optically active Δ^1-THC it seems that the synthesis reported by Petrzilka and that of our group are the methods of choice. Preference for either route depends on the local availability of terpenoid starting material (verbenol in our synthesis and p-menthadien 2,8-01-1 in the Swiss synthesis).

It is worthwhile pointing out that all syntheses use olivetol, the preparation of which is quite tedious and is probably beyond the capability of an illegal laboratory. Hence, if the appropriate government agencies take steps to ensure that olivetol and related materials

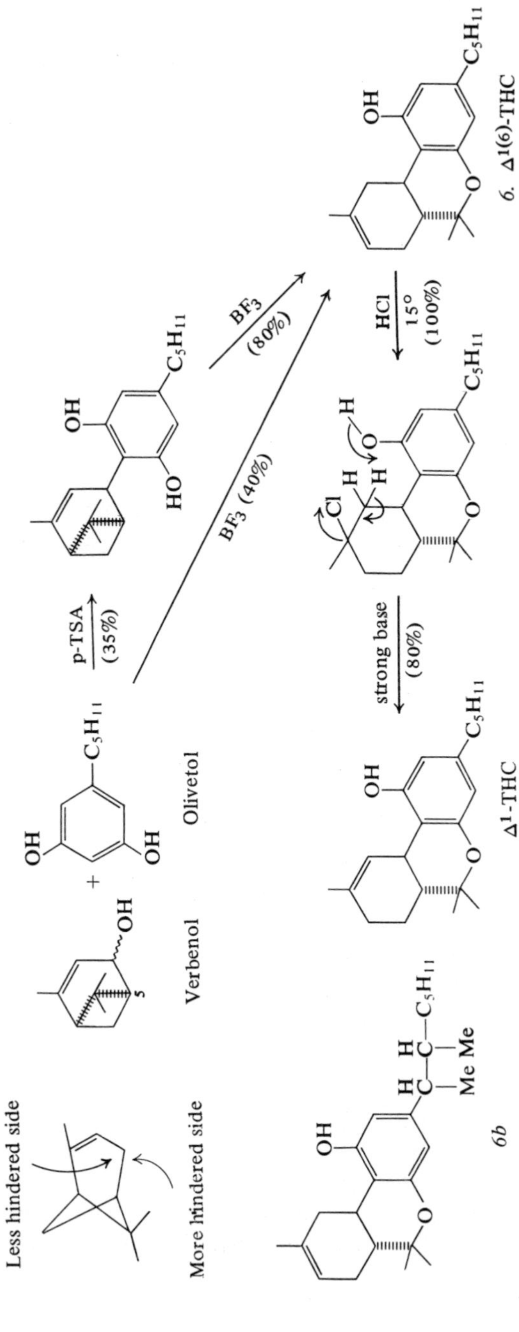
Less hindered side
More hindered side
6b
Me Me
Verbenol
Olivetol
p-TSA
(35%)
BF3 (40%)
BF3
(80%)
6. Δ1(6)-THC
HCl
15°
(100%)
strong base
(80%)
Δ1-THC

Scheme 5.

remain commercially non-available, active THC isomers will not become illegally available. On the other hand the relatively easy syntheses of Δ^1-THC now make possible a thorough investigation of the hashish problem.

We have employed our synthetic route in the preparation of a number of THC analogues, some of which were tested on monkeys. We have not found any striking increase of activity as compared to the natural THC derivatives. The most active material so far seems to be the dimethylheptyl analogue *6b,* which is several times as active as $\Delta^{1(6)}$-THC (*6*).

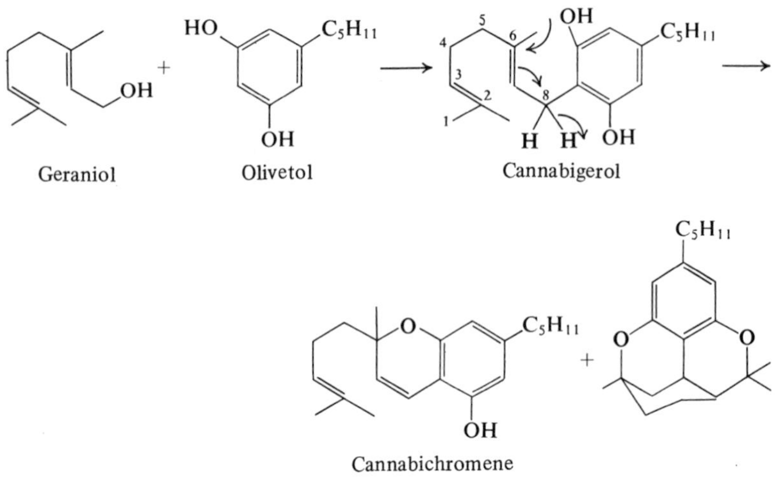

Geraniol   Olivetol   Cannabigerol

Cannabichromene

Scheme 6.

With the successful completion of this phase of our synthetic work we turned our attention to the other natural cannabinoids. We consider this endeavour of interest not only as an academic exercise but as a study of a more general nature. It is not yet known whether the other natural cannabinoids, which are inactive *per se,* influence the activity of Δ^1-THC. There are grounds to believe that this may indeed be the case. Habitués believe that hashish samples of different origin show more than quantitative differences. Thus Afghanistan hashish is supposed to cause euphoria exclusively while Lebanese hashish may on occasion induce depression. We do not know any data which support or disprove such claims. The availability of pure synthetic constituents should now make possible research in this area.

Cannabigerol was prepared in 40% yield, by the condensation of geraniol and olivetol with p-toluene sulphonic acid in methylene chloride (Gaoni and Mechoulam, 1964a; Mechoulam and Yagen, 1969). The synthesis of cannabichromene* was achieved by dehydrogenation of cannabigerol with chloranil (Mechoulam, Yagnitinsky and Gaoni, 1968).

This reaction probably proceeds via hydride abstraction from C_8, as shown in the scheme opposite. Cardillo, Cricchio and Merlini (1968) have suggested a different mechanism, involving the formation of an o-quinone methide.

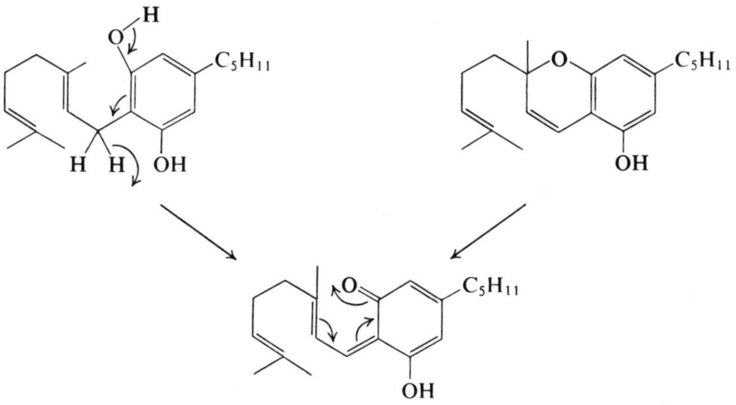

Scheme 7.

While in the case of cannabigerol this point is as yet unsettled, in the THC series the phenolic group apparently does not participate in the reaction. Dehydrogenation with chloranil of both Δ^1-THC and Δ^1-THC acetate proceeds at about the same rate, though obviously in the case of the acetate it cannot take place via the ketonic intermediate.

---

* Synthetic cannabichromene was inactive in the ataxia or monkey behaviour tests. We had previously reported that the natural material was active (Gaoni and Mechoulam, 1966a). This was apparently due to contamination, and has now been disproved.

From a biogenetic point of view, if the symmetrical o-quinone methide intermediate is involved in the formation of natural cannabichromene then one can understand the lack of optical activity in both cannabichromene and cannabicyclol.

There are subtle stereoelectronic factors which govern the chloranil dehydrogenations in the cannabinoid series. We have established that in contrast to Δ^1-THC (*4*), Δ^1-cis-THC (*11*) and cannabidiol (*2a*) remain unchanged on dehydrogenation under identical experimental conditions. We have explained these observations as follows.

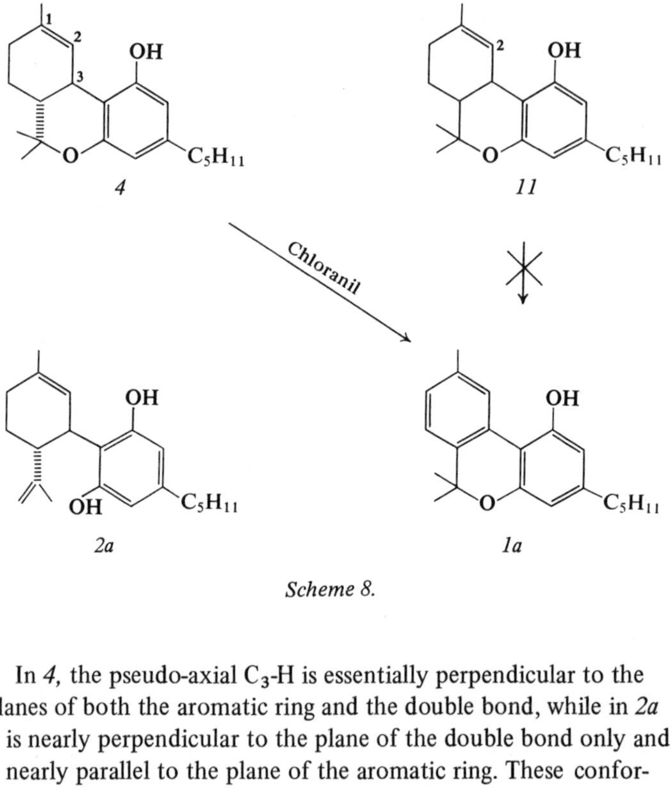

Scheme 8.

In *4*, the pseudo-axial C_3-H is essentially perpendicular to the planes of both the aromatic ring and the double bond, while in *2a* it is nearly perpendicular to the plane of the double bond only and is nearly parallel to the plane of the aromatic ring. These conformations have been deduced from NMR analysis.

In *4*, the C_3-H, during abstraction as the hydride, will remain in constant overlap with the π electrons of both unsaturated systems, thus lowering the energy of the transition state. In *2a* overlap is possible with the π electrons of the double bond only. The same factors are probably involved in the non-reactivity of *11*. The C_2-H in the preferred conformation of *11* is at a dihedral angle of *ca.* 35° with the C_3-H and hence σ-π overlap in the transition state is limited to the phenolic ring only, with which C_3-H forms an angle of *ca.* 80°.

A major group of cannabinoids which had until recently eluded synthesis are the cannabinoid acids. This was probably due to the fact

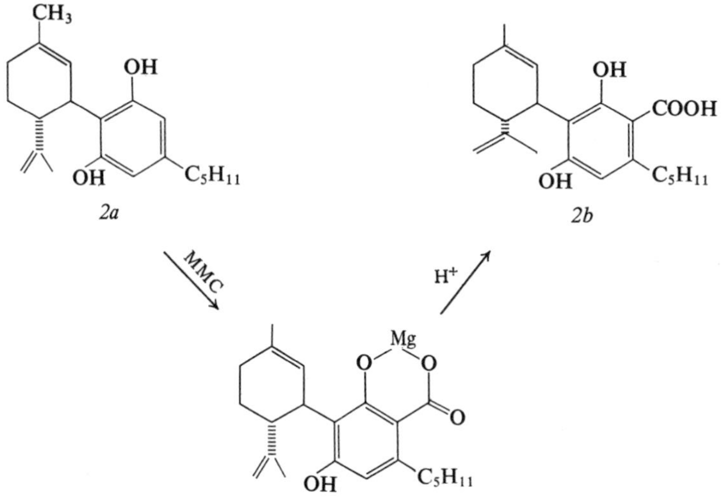

MMC = CH₃OMgOCO(OMe)

Scheme 9.

that the **Kolbe-Schmidt** reaction, which is the standard method for the preparation of phenolic acids does not convert non-acidic cannabinoids into the corresponding acids (under the ordinary conditions for this reaction). We reported recently the first synthesis of some of these acids via a new synthetic method (Mechoulam and Ben-Zvi, 1969). The method is based on the use of magnesium methyl carbonate (MMC), a reagent employed for the carboxylation of ketones, nitroalkanes and related compounds possessing an acidic hydrogen (Stiles, 1959; Stiles and Finkbeiner, 1959; Stiles, 1960; Finkbeiner and Stiles, 1963; Finkbeiner, 1965; Finkbeiner, 1966; Crombie, Hemesley and Pattenden, 1968). This reaction has not been used up till now in aromatic substitutions. The easy hydrogen-deuterium exchange in positions *ortho-* and *para-* to the hydroxyl groups in the resorcinol series in weakly alkaline solutions suggests that these hydrogens are acidic (Hand and Horowitz, 1966). This observation led us to investigate the possible selective carboxylation of resorcinols with MMC. Indeed when MMC reacted with this group of compounds mono- and di-carboxylic acids were obtained. Other phenolic types did not react. When applied to the cannabinoids we found that it was possible to obtain cannabidiolic acid (*2b*) from cannabidiol (*2a*) in 96% yield, cannabigerolic acid (*3b*) from cannabigerol (*3a*) in 78% yield and Δ^1-THC acid A (*7a*) from Δ^1-THC (*4*) in about 9% yield, the rest being mostly starting material. The easy separation of product (an acid) and starting material allows a considerable increase in the yield of Δ^1-THC acid by a recycling process.

With the completion of these syntheses most of the natural cannabinoids are now easily available. It should be possible, through collaboration of chemists and biologists, to make rapid advances in all areas of cannabinoid research.

ANALYTICAL ASPECTS: THE BEAM TEST

An amusing curiosity of cannabinoid analysis is that the most widely used colour test for the identification of hashish is based on the

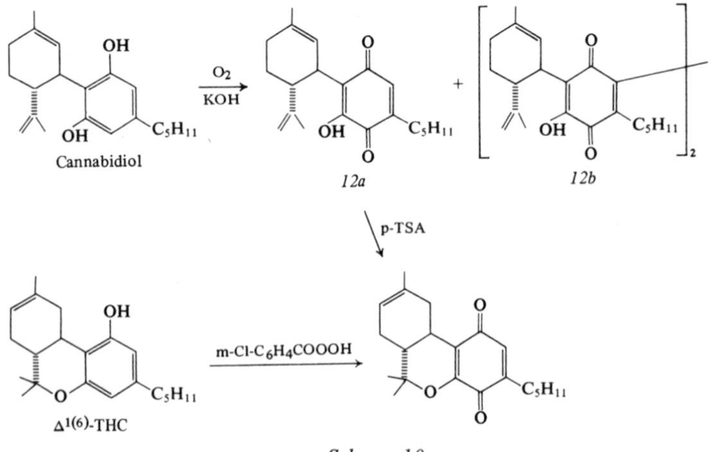

Scheme 10.

presence of the inactive constituents cannabidiol (*2a*) and cannabigerol (*3a*) (and the corresponding acids).

Beam (1911) reported from Khartoum that hashish extracts gave a deep purple colour with a 5% ethanolic potassium hydroxide solution. In view of the considerable importance of cannabis identification for legal purposes this test has been the object of numerous studies as regards its specificity, reliability and sensitivity (Grlić, 1964). However, the chemical basis of this reaction has remained unknown. We have now found (Mechoulam, Ben-Zvi and Gaoni, 1968) that under the reaction conditions of the Beam test cannabidiol is oxidized to the monomeric quinone *12a* and the dimeric quinone *12b*. The violet colour is due to the anions of these hydroxy quinones. The quinone *12a* has been correlated with an oxidation product of $\Delta^{1(6)}$-THC.

The cannabinoids being phenolic are prone to give coloured products. Thus Δ^{1}-THC after chromatography acquires a violet tinge. The active oily extract of marihuana is red; on prolonged exposure to air it turns dark. A petroleum ether solution of Δ^{3}-THC after chromatography is blue (unpublished data). The nature of these coloured products is as yet unknown.

Cyclizations and isomerizations in the cannabinoid series

The presence of numerous double bonds and free phenolic groups in the molecules of most cannabinoids makes them labile to acids (Gaoni and Mechoulam, 1966a; Gaoni and Mechoulam, 1966b; Gaoni and Mechoulam, 1968; Yagen and Mechoulam, 1969). In the following schemes some of the cyclizations observed are described. For purposes of classification we have named "iso-tetrahydrocannabinols" those THC isomers in which the etheric linkage is attached to C_1.

Reaction of geraniol with olivetol gives cannabigerol (*3a*) while that of nerol with olivetol yields 6-*cis*-cannabigerol (*13*). Cyclization of *3a* with 100% sulphuric acid in methylene chloride at $-30°$ gives the *trans*-tricyclic chromane *14*, while *13* gives mainly the *cis*-tricyclic chromane *15*. In both cases negligible amounts of the bicyclic *16* are also obtained (Mechoulam and Yagen, 1969). These results are in accordance with the Stork-Eschenmoser hypothesis that the stereochemical course of cyclizations of acyclic polyenes induced by acid is dictated by the configuration of the central double bond (Johnson,

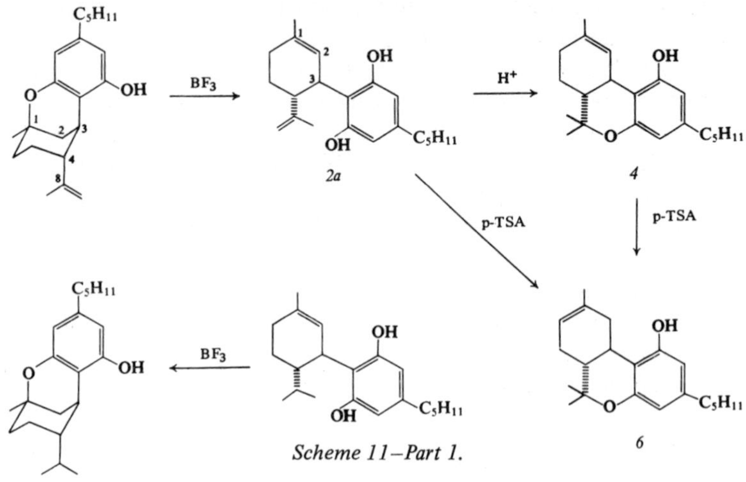

Scheme 11—Part 1.

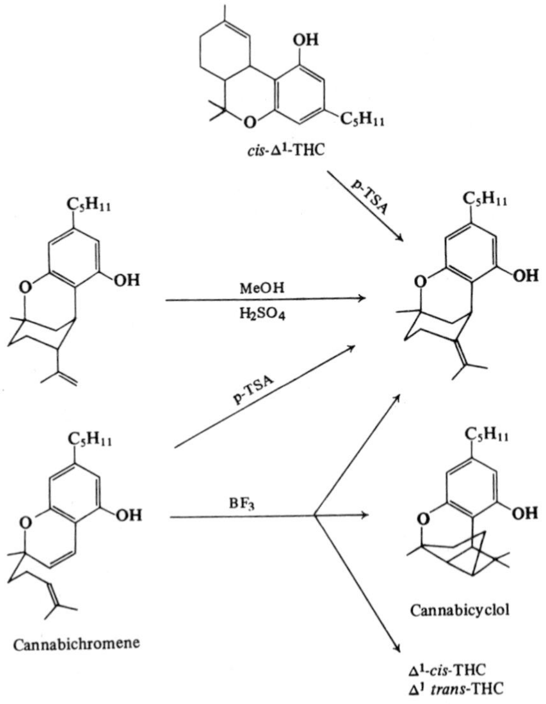

Scheme 11—Part 2.

1968). The stereo-specificity demands either a concerted mechanism
or cationic intermediates which maintain the stereochemical integrity.
As the temperature is increased the stereospecificity decreases and the
amount of the bicyclic *16* increases. At 80° both *3a* and *13* give mainly
16, and, unexpectedly, the *cis*-tricyclic chromane *15.* By contrast when
the cyclization is performed in benzene with p-toluene sulphonic acid
both *3* and *13* give mainly *16* and the *trans*-tricyclic chromane *14.*
These results indicate an intricate interplay of conformational and
electronic factors.

METABOLISM OF THE TETRAHYDROCANNABINOLS

Recently Dr. S. Burstein* of the Worcester Foundation in Massachusetts in collaboration with our group initiated a programme aimed
at elucidating the metabolism of the tetrahydrocannabinols. For this
purpose $\Delta^{1(6)}$-THC was stereo-specifically labelled with tritium at C_2
(Burstein and Mechoulam, 1968).

The metabolism of $\Delta^{1(6)}$-THC-$2H^3$ was examined in the rabbit
both *in vivo* and *in vitro.* The preliminary findings indicated that
when the material is injected intravenously it is metabolized and
excreted in the urine at the rate of 1-2% per day. In liver perfusion
studies and in incubations with liver homogenates the compound
is rapidly converted to several metabolites. All of the metabolites
(urinary and *in vitro*) give rise to one common product when treated
with mineral acid. The evidence to date suggests that its formula
is that shown in *17,* for the following reasons: (1) the mass spectrum
of the diacetate, which has the correct molecular ion peak and peaks
for M^+-C_2H_2O and M^+-CH_3COOH, is consistent with *17;* (2) oxidation
with DDQ, showing that the aliphatic hydroxyl is allylic; and (3) conversion to cannabinol by acid treatment showing that the carbon
skeleton is not altered during metabolism or isolation (Burstein,
Menezes, Williamson and Mechoulam, 1970).

* The work at Worcester was carried out with the able assistance of Dr.
Franco Menezes and Mrs. Ethel Williamson. The support of this work by the
NIMH (Grant No. MH 16051) is gratefully acknowledged. We also would like
to acknowledge the contribution of Dr. William Dawson of the Worcester
Foundation who performed the liver perfusion.

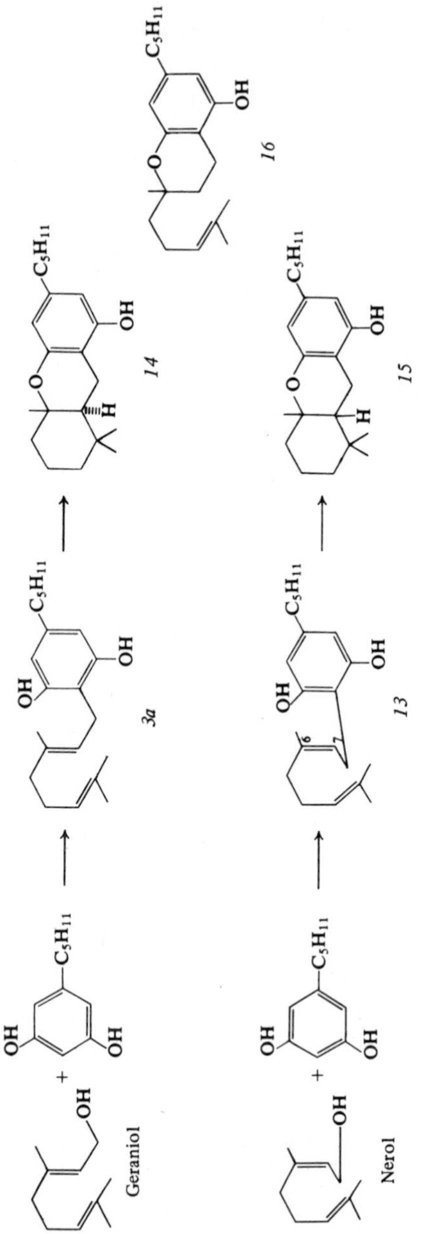

Scheme 12.

Recent work has confirmed structure 17 by direct comparison with synthetic material (Mechoulam, Ben-Zvi and Burstein, 1970). Experiments are also being carried out to elucidate the nature of the conjugates.

Further attempts at labelling with C^{14} and H^3 are in progress both with $\Delta^{1(6)}$-THC and with Δ^1-THC.

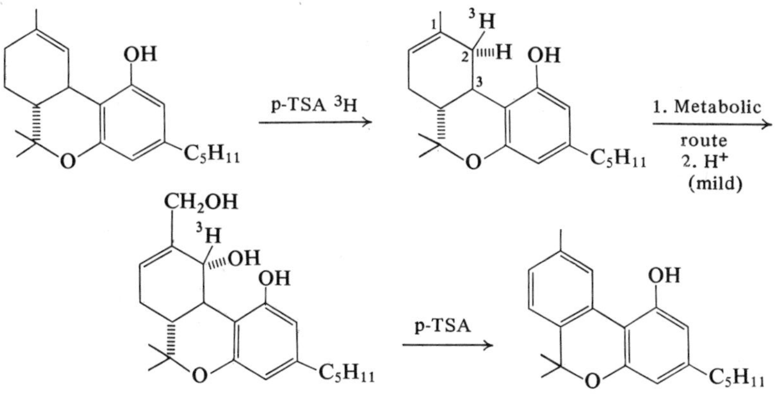

Scheme 13.

In addition to the intrinsic interest in and importance of metabolic and biochemical work in this field, this research may lead to the isolation of metabolites which could serve for the identification of cannabis in body fluids. At present there are no generally accepted tests for this (see, however, da Silva, 1967).

As the metabolism of Δ^1-THC follows a parallel metabolic route (Wall, Brine, Brine, Pitt, Freudenthal and Christensen, 1970), it can be assumed that a relatively simple forensic test can be developed. Acid treatment of the metabolites will cleave the conjugates and cause dehydration, followed by dehydration, thus leading to cannabinol. The major problem will probably be to find a method sensitive enough to detect the minute amounts of cannabinol that are formed.

PHOTOCHEMISTRY OF THE CANNABINOIDS

We have observed a number of photochemical reactions in the cannabinoid series. The cyclization of cannabichromene to cannabicyclol has been mentioned (Crombie *et al.,* 1968). Some other reactions are as follows (unpublished data):

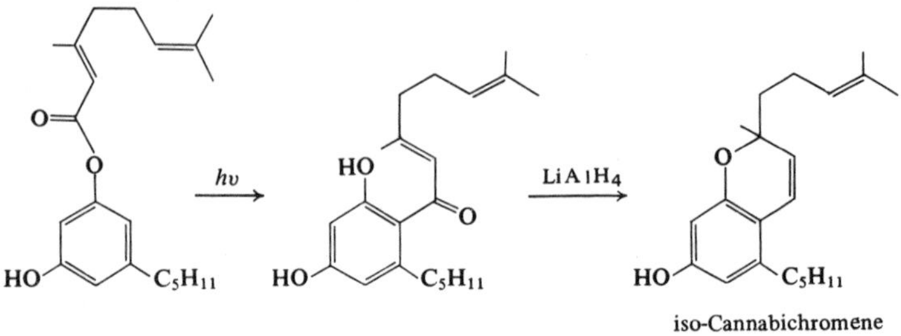

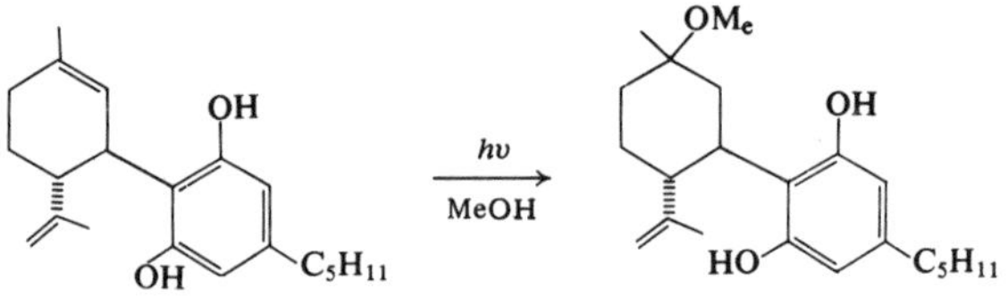

iso-Cannabichromene

QUO VADIMUS?

Predictions as to the paths a branch of science will follow partake somewhat of the nature of crystal-gazing. And yet in the proceedings of a symposium aimed at delineating future research we must try to put down some of the obvious developments:

1. **Synthetic modifications of cannabinoid molecules**

   In view of the diverse, pharmacologically interesting activities exhibited by this class of compounds such as analgesia, antibiotic activity, euphoria etc., we expect to see a certain amount of experimental therapeutic work, especially by the pharmaceutical houses.

2. **The use of cannabinoids as models in the investigation of organic reactions.**

   The considerable variety of closely related cannabinoids makes possible the use of this class of compounds in investigations in the field of stereochemistry, intramolecular reactions, and reaction mechanisms in general. As described above, we have already made use of the cannabinoids in investigations on the mechanism of chloranil dehydrogenations, polyolefinic cyclizations etc.

3. **Synthesis of labelled cannabinoids for metabolic and pharmacologic studies.**

4. **Pharmacological and clinical studies.**
   The ready availability of synthetic cannabinoids should make possible fast advances in these fields.

5. **The mode of action of cannabinoids at the molecular level**
   This virgin area of research can become a most fascinating and important field of future molecular biology.

Acknowledgement   Some of the research reported here was made possible by a NIMH grant (No. MH 13180) for which we are grateful. We are indebted to the Israeli Police for the supply of hashish.

References

Beam, W., Fourth Report Wellcome Tropical Research Lab. Chem. Sect., Khartoum, B25 (1911); *Ibid.* Bulletin No. 3 (1915).

Bicher, J. I. and Mechoulam, R., *Arch. Intern. Pharmacodyn.* 172:24 (1968).

Burstein, S. and Mechoulam, R., *J. Am. Chem. Soc.* 90:2420 (1968).

Burstein, S. H., Menezes, F., Williamson, E. and Mechoulam, R., *Nature,* 225:87 (1970).

Cardillo, G., Cricchio, R. and Merlini, L., *Tetrahedron,* 24:4825 (1968).

Claussen, U. and Korte, F., *Ann.* 713:162 (1968).

Claussen, U., von Spulak, F. and Korte, F., *Tetrahedron,* 22:1477 (1966).

Claussen, U., von Spulak, F. and Korte, F., *Tetrahedron,* 24:1021 (1968).

Crombie, L., Hemesley, P. and Pattenden, G., *Tet. Letters,* 3021 (1968).

Crombie, L. and Ponsford, R., *Tet. Letters,* 894, 4557 (1968).

Crombie, L., Ponsford, R., Shani, A., Yagnitinsky, B. and Mechoulam, R., *Tet. Letters,* 5771 (1968).

Finkbeiner, H. L., *J. Am. Chem. Soc.* 87:4588, (1965).

Finkbeiner, H. L., *J. Org. Chem.* 30:1747 (1966).

Finkbeiner, H. L. and Stiles, M., *J. Am. Chem. Soc.* 85:616 (1963).

Gaoni, Y. and Mechoulam, R., *Proc. Chem. Soc.* 82 (1964a).

Gaoni, Y. and Mechoulam, R., *J. Am. Chem. Soc.* 86:1646 (1964b).

Gaoni, Y. and Mechoulam, R., *Chem. Commun.* 20 (1966a).

Gaoni, Y. and Mechoulam, R., *Tetrahedron*, 22:1481 (1966b).

Gaoni, Y. and Mechoulam, R., *J. Am. Chem. Soc.* 88:5673 (1966c).

Gaoni, Y. and Mechoulam, R., *Isr. J. Chem.* 6:679 (1968).

Grlić, L., *Bull. Narcotics*, 16:29 (1964).

Grunfeld, Y. and Edery, H., *Psychopharmacologia*, 14:200 (1969).

Hand, E. S. and Horowitz, R. M., *J. Am. Chem. Soc.* 86:2084 (1966).

Hively, R. L., Mosher, W. A. and Hoffmann, F. W., *J. Am. Chem. Soc.* 88:1832 (1966).

Isbell, H., Gorodetsky, C. W., Jasinski, D., Claussen, U., von Spulak, F. and Korte, F., *Psychopharmacologia*, 11:184 (1967).

Jen, T. Y., Hughes, G. A. and Smith, H., *J. Am. Chem. Soc.* 89:4551 (1967).

Johnson, W. S., *Accounts Chem. Research*, 1:1 (1968).

Kane, V. V. and Razdan, R. K., *J. Am. Chem. Soc.* 90:6551 (1968).

Korte, F., Haag, M. and Claussen, U., *Angew. Chem.* (Intern. Ed.) 4:872 (1965).

Lerner, M. and Zeffert, J. T., *Bull. Narcotics*, 20(2):53, (1968).

Mechoulam, R. and Ben-Zvi, Z., *Chem. Commun.* 343 (1969).

Mechoulam, R., Ben-Zvi, Z. and Burstein, S., *J. Am. Chem. Soc.* 92:3468 (1970).

Mechoulam, R., Ben-Zvi, Z. and Gaoni, Y., *Tetrahedron*, 24:5615 (1968).

Mechoulam, R., Ben-Zvi, Z., Yagnitinsky, B. and Shani, A., *Tet. Letters*, 2339 (1969).

Mechoulam, R., Braun, P. and Gaoni, Y., *J. Am. Chem. Soc.* 89:4552 (1967).

Mechoulam, R. and Gaoni, Y., *Tetrahedron*, 21:1223 (1965a).

Mechoulam, R. and Gaoni, Y., *J. Am. Chem. Soc.* 87:3273 (1965b).

Mechoulam, R. and Gaoni, Y., *Fortschr. Chem. Organ, Naturstoffe*, 25:175 (1967a).

Mechoulam, R. and Gaoni, Y., *Tet. Letters*, 1109 (1967b).

Mechoulam, R. and Shvo, Y., *Tetrahedron*, 19:2073 (1963).

Mechoulam, R. and Yagen, B., *Tet. Letters*, 5349 (1969).

Mechoulam, R., Yagnitinsky, B. and Gaoni, Y., *J. Am. Chem. Soc.* 90:2418 (1968).

Nilsson, I. M., Agurell, S., Nilsson, J. L. G., Ohlsson, A. Sandberg, F. and Wahlqvist, M. *Science* 168: 1228 (1970).

Petrzilka, T. and Sikemeier, C., *Helv. Chim. Acta.* 50:2111 (1967a).

Petrzilka, T. and Sikemeier, C., *Helv. Chim. Acta.* 50:1416 (1967b).

Petrzilka, T., Haefliger, W., Sikemeier, C., Ohloff, G. and Eschenmoser, A., *Helv. Chim. Acta.* 50:719 (1967).

da Silva, J. B., *Rev. Fac. Farm. Bioquim. S. Paulo*, 5:205 (1967).

Stiles, M., *J. Am. Chem. Soc.* 81:2598 (1959).

Stiles, M., *Ann. New York Acad. Sci.* 88:332 (1960).

Stiles, M. and Finkbeiner, H. L. *J. Am. Chem. Soc.* 81:505 (1959).

Taylor, E. C., Lenard, K. and Shvo, Y., *J. Am. Chem. Soc.* 88:367 (1967).

U. N. Econ. Social Council, Comm. Narcotic Drugs, Document E-CN, 7-479 (1965).

Wall, M. E., Brine, D. R., Brine, G. A., Pitt, C. G., Freudenthal, R. I. and Christensen, H. D., *J. Am. Chem. Soc.* 92:3466 (1970).

Weil, A. E., Zinberg, N. E. and Nelson, J. M., *Science,* 162:1234 (1968).

Wollner, H. J., Matchett, J. R., Levine, J. and Loewe, S., *J. Am. Chem. Soc.* 64:26 (1942).

Wolstenholme, G. E. and Knight, J. (Ed.), "Hashish: Its Chemistry and Pharmacology," Churchill, London, 1965.

Yagen, B. and Mechoulam, R., *Tet. Letters,* 5353 (1969).

Yamauchi, T., Shoyama, Y., Aramaki, H., Azuma, T. and Nishioka, I., *Chem. Pharm. Bull.* 15:1075 (1967).

3 Recent Results in Hashish Chemistry

F. Korte

The interest of my group in hashish arose out of a general interest in chemical classification of plants. We therefore commenced an investigation of hashish from plants of *Cannabis sativa* grown in warm climates, and in Central Europe. These will be referred to subsequently as *"indica"* and *"non-indica"*, respectively (but see Part One of the present volume).

Comparison of Cannabis sativa indica and Cannabis sativa non-indica
From 1956 onwards, we have cultivated plants from both sources, under identical conditions, and have isolated oils from them. However, the constituents of these oils are rather unstable, and although they can be separated by thin layer chromatography, isolation by conventional methods fails. Therefore we have used counter-current distribution techniques (O'Keefe method). Fig. 1 shows the curves of counter-current distribution. The O'Keefe method permits counter-current distribution of the upper and lower phase, while keeping one compound in the machine by adjusting the process to a known distribution coefficient. The mixture of compounds is introduced into the centre of the machine; compounds with a higher distribution coefficient are removed by the upper phase, and those with a lower coefficient are removed by the lower phase. This method is very convenient for concentrating substances available only in small amounts. Furthermore, the apparatus permits the use of extremely mild conditions, such as an inert gas atmosphere, complete darkness, etc. When several thousand transfers have been made, which takes at least 6 to 7 weeks, a few milligrams are isolated and attempts can be made to elucidate the structure.

Once reliable analytical methods had been found, we again cultivated Cannabis from both sources and worked them up in the normal
manner, without taking into consideration whether the products were
artefacts or not. In extracts of *Cannabis indica* and *Cannabis non indica*
grown in Germany we found cannabidiol as well as the active hashish
principle tetrahydrocannabinol. The ratio of active hashish compounds
in *Cannabis indica* and *Cannabis non indica* was about 10:1.

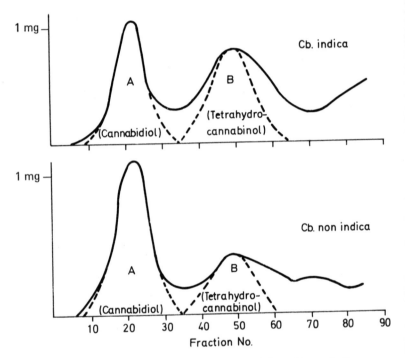

Fig. 1. Craig-partition of Cannabis indica and Cannabis non-indica
after chromatography on Al_2O_3.

Hashish is not a plant constituent, but either a resinous material
which the plant produces after efflorescence on the flowering tops
of the female plant. Fig. 2 gives a survey of the present state of our
knowledge about the active principle. The compound shown is *trans*-
9,10-tetrahydrocannabinol. It has now been isolated with a uniform
optical rotation value, almost simultaneously, by Mechoulam and his
colleagues in Israel and by our team. Despite the very different

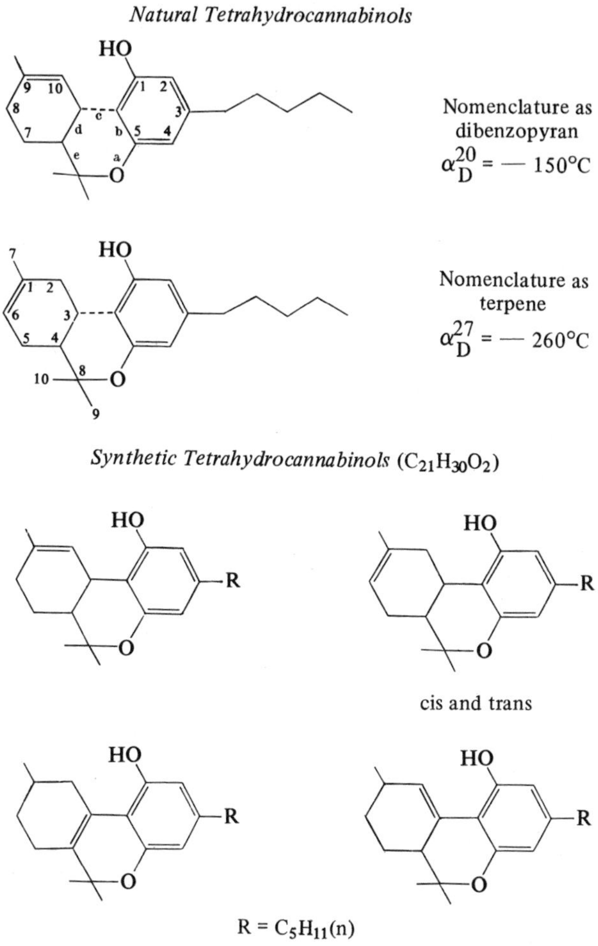

Natural Tetrahydrocannabinols

Nomenclature as
dibenzopyran
$\alpha_D^{20} = -150°C$

Nomenclature as
terpene
$\alpha_D^{27} = -260°C$

Synthetic Tetrahydrocannabinols ($C_{21}H_{30}O_2$)

cis and trans

$R = C_5H_{11}(n)$

Fig. 2. Natural and synthetic tetrahydrocannabinols.

nomenclatures employed, the only important fact is that in the natural tetrahydrocannabinol, the double bond is in the 9,10-position; the strokes are methyl groups and the substituent at the nucleus is a n-pentyl group. According to private information, Hoffmann has isolated another compound as a natural tetrahydrocannabinol; he has found that in small samples the double bond may also be in the 1,6 or 8,9-position.

PHARMACOLOGY

We were interested to find out whether the tetrahydrocannabinol known in 1954 (this was certainly not a uniform compound) was responsible for the activity. We contacted a considerable number of pharmacologists in order to find efficient test methods. However, all tests available proved unsatisfactory; at the time the ataxia test with dogs was considered to be the best method. Some years ago we heard of Dr. Harris Isbell of the Drug Addiction Research Centre in Lexington,

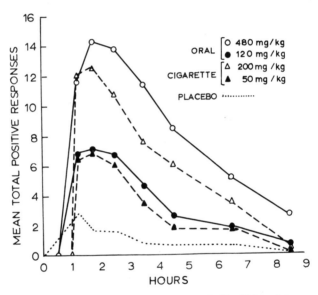

Fig. 3. Relative response to oral and smoked hashish, and to placebo.

Kentucky, who has facilities for testing compounds on humans. This constitutes an enormous advantage; the values obtained in these tests are exact and reproducible, and our work has made notable progress while collaborating with Dr. Isbell. Fig. 3 summarises results from some of the tests carried out by Dr. Isbell and his co-workers. To a certain group of test persons the extract with known amounts of tetrahydrocannabinol, or the pure compound, were given orally. The following observations were made one hour before the drug was given and one, two, three, five, seven, nine and eleven hours after following bed rest for ten minutes: rectal temperature, systolic and diastolic blood pressures and respiratory rate. In addition, pulse rate and systolic blood pressure were determined after standing quietly for one minute.

The subjective effects of the drug were assessed by administration of a special questionnaire consisting of thirty-one questions. The

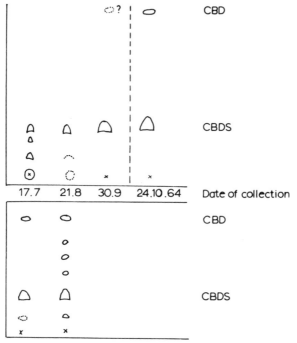

The same extracts as above, after concentration at 30°C and storage at 0°C.

Fig. 4. Thin layer chromatograms of hashish extracts.

questionnaire was completed by the patient with the help of an aide at the following times: ½ hour before the drug, 1½ hours, 2½ hours, 3½ hours, 5½ hours, 7½ hours, 9½ hours and 11½ hours after the drug. The questions included "drug similarity" items such as: is it like LSD? is it like heroin? is it like "reefer" (marihuana)? etc. The questions also dealt with mood, e.g.: is your hearing keen? are colours brighter? does time pass slowly? etc. There were also questions dealing with thinking and questions concerning delusions, hallucinations etc.

These tests showed that the activity paralleled the tetrahydro-cannabinol content of the extract. They give an indication of which is the active hashish principle and we can now say that analytical grade tetrahydrocannabinol shows about 70% of the activity of the tetrahydrocannabinol in the crude extract. So far, we have not determined whether this is due to a synergistic or to a resorption effect. It is certain, however, that none of the other cannabis products isolated as a pure compound has shown much activity, resembling that of hashish. Thus we can safely state that Δ^9-tetrahydrocannabinol must be mainly responsible for the activity of hashish.

To determine if the active hashish component might be an artificial product, we investigated the substances produced by Cannabis plants during the vegetation period. In all plants studied, we only found cannabidiol carboxylic acid (CBDS) and other compounds of strong polarity but no compound of low polarity (Fig. 4). Therefore it can be concluded that neither tetrahydrocannabinol nor cannabidiol were to be found in the growing plant. After the period of growth, the plants were harvested and worked up. Then we found cannabidiol, which was probably formed by decarboxylation of cannabidiol carboxylic acid. However, we have no idea whether this was effected enzymatically or not. When these extracts were evaporated at $30°C$, and stored at $0°C$, only cannabidiol and its carboxylic acid were found from which we concluded that cannabidiol is an artificial product not present in the fresh plant (see Fig. 4).

ANALYTICAL METHODS

Table 1 shows reagents which have been used for detection on TLC. All known colour reagents proved unsatisfactory, because they were neither sensitive nor specific enough for our purposes. However, Echtblausalz Merck (Di-o-anisidine tetrazolium chloride) enabled cannabidiol (orange), cannabinol (violet), and tetrahydrocannabinol (red) to be distinguished on thin layer chromatograms.

In speaking of "tetrahydrocannabinols" we must remember that the only analytical method available at the time of this work was thin layer chromatography. We could only evaluate the R_f value and the colour of a spot. Nevertheless the use of Echtblausalz had the advantage of the colour as an extra criterion.

TABLE 1. *Colour reactions of cannobinols after thin layer chromatography*

Reagent	colour and visibility frontier (μg)		
	CBD	CBN	THC
Gibbs reagent (2,6 dibromquinone-4-chlorimide-iso-propylamine)	Blue-green 1	Blue-green 1	Grey-violet 1
Ghamrawy reagent (p-dimethylamino-benzaldehyde-H_2SO_4)	Brownish-red 0.5	Brownish-red 1	Brownish-red 1
Duquenois reagent (vanillin-acet-aldehyde-HCl)	Violet 0.5	Violet 10	Violet 1
Blackie reagent (benzaldehyde-iso-butanol)	No colour	No colour	No colour
Beam reagent (5% ethanolic KOH)	0.5	No colour	No colour
Echtblausalz (Merck) (di-o-anisidine-tetrazolium-chloride)	Colour 0.01	Violet 0.01	Red 0.01

CBD = Cannabidiol
CBN = Cannabinol
THC = Tetrahydrocannabinol

TABLE 2. *Content of cannabinolic compounds in cannabis-extracts (UN seizure)*

	% of dry drug		
	CBD	THC	CBN
Nigeria UNC 59	–	0.098	0.481
Brasil UNC 61	–	0.190	0.410
Cyprus UNC 33	–	0.380	0.060
Marocco UNC 21	0.129	0.096	0.123
Geneva UNC 51	0.129	0.087	0.017
Canada UNC 37	0.103	traces	–

CBD = Cannabidiol
THC = Tetrahydrocannabinol
CBN = Cannabinol

Thin layer chromatograms of extracts of Cannabis plants cultivated in Germany, as well as of hashish samples of different origin (obtained from the Federal German Criminal Investigation Office and the Narcotics Division of W.H.O.), showed not one, but three "tetrahydrocannabinols" (Fig. 5). We called these compounds tetrahydrocannabinol isomers I, II, III at that time. Cannabinol, that is the dehydrogenation product, was found only in hashish samples. Cannabidiol as well as its carboxylic acid were found in plant extracts and hashish samples. It was remarkable that on all thin layer chromatograms the hashish samples gave a greater number of phenolic compounds than the plant

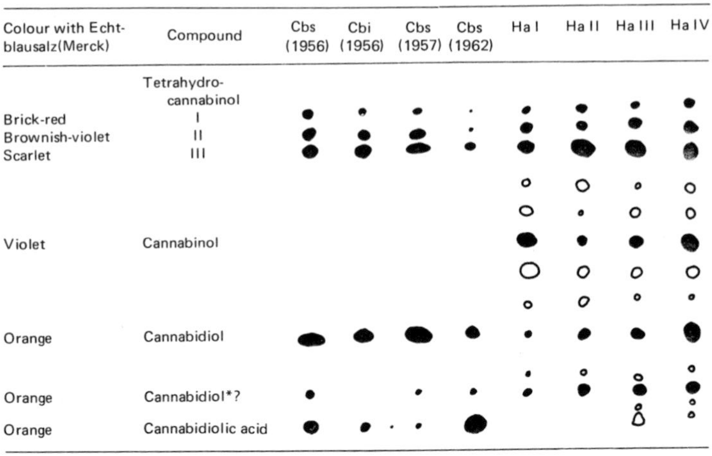

Colour with Echtblausalz(Merck)	Compound	Cbs (1956)	Cbi (1956)	Cbs (1957)	Cbs (1962)	Ha I	Ha II	Ha III	Ha IV
	Tetrahydrocannabinol								
Brick-red	I								
Brownish-violet	II								
Scarlet	III								
Violet	Cannabinol								
Orange	Cannabidiol								
Orange	Cannabidiol*?								
Orange	Cannabidiolic acid								

Fig. 5. Thin layer chromatograms of hashish extracts.

extracts. We tested a number of hashish samples for their tetrahydrocannabinol content, which varied considerably (Table 2).

We next isolated the three different tetrahydrocannabinols that we had found to vary in concentration in hashish samples and in plant extracts. Thin layer chromatography is an extremely sensitive qualitative method which is difficult to handle quantitatively. We therefore developed methods of gas-chromatography analysis which is less sensitive but easier to perform quantitatively. So we can now separate the different hashish compounds—cannabigerol, cannabinol, cannabidiol, tetrahydrocannabinol and cannabidiolic acid by gas chromatography in one step in a Golay column (Fig. 6).

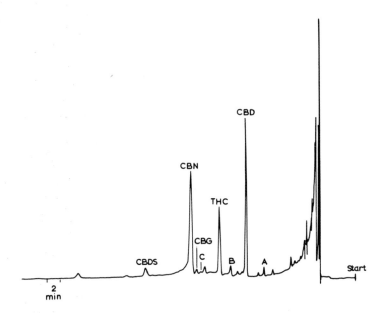

Fig. 6. Gas chromatogram of certain cannabinoids. (G.L.C. conditions: Golay column SE 30, 50 m; 0.25 mm φ steel; F 6/4 HF; 1.5 ml He/min; 240°C; volume 2 μl; stream splitting 1:7.8; FID. Relative retention volumes: A 0.63; B. 1.19; $\Delta^{9,10}$ THC 1.35; Δ^{d}THC 1.44; C 1.54; CBG 1.60; $\Delta^{10,10a}$THC 1.63; CBN 1.72; CBC 2.04; CBDS (CBDA) 2.44; CBD 1.00. Abbreviations: CBD Cannabidiol; THC Tetrahydrocannabidiol; CBN Cannabinol; CBDS Cannabidiolic acid; A,B,C Frequently occurring previously unknown substances; CBG Cannabigerol; compounds chromatographed as TMS ethers.)

STRUCTURE OF SOME PHENOLIC HASHISH CONSTITUENTS

We were able to show that tetrahydrocannabinol II is a chromene, which we called cannabichromene. Its constitution was determined by a combination of IR, UV, NMR and mass spectrometry (Fig. 7), and only this formula is in agreement with the data obtained.

Mechoulam in Israel and my group in Germany worked simultaneously on the isolation of cannabichromene, without any knowledge of the other team's investigations. Our paper on this compound was received on 15th November 1965 and his 8 days later on the 23rd! We not only furnished the same evidence, but independently of each other even proposed the same name for this compound, really an extraordinary coincidence.

The power of modern analytical methods is shown by the identification of cannabichromene. The AB-spectrum of protons D and E show the remarkable difference of chemical shift which only can be explained by the chromene structure. Protons H and I show two distinct signals, owing to the different shielding caused by the neighbourhood of the ether oxygen and the hydroxyl oxygen respectively. These signals coincide if a complex is formed. We isolated the tetrahydrocannabinol carboxylic acid as a complex with dimethylformamide.

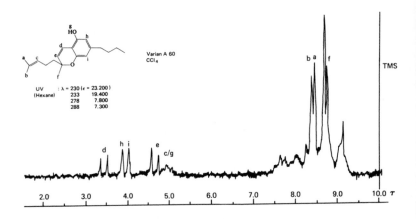

Fig. 7. NMR spectrum of tetrahydrocannabinol II.

If such a complex with tetrahydrocannabinol is formed, the two signals coincide in the NMR-spectrum due to identical shielding. Thus we were able to show that tetrahydrocannabinol II, isolated by the same method, has not the same structure as tetrahydrocannabinol, though it gives similar RF-values in thin layer chromatography. Now we turn to mass spectrometry. About 18 months ago, the Budzikiewicz group investigated the products obtained by Mechoulam and his co-workers, but their results did not agree with ours. The explanation of this disagreement is uncertain. Either the double bonds in Mechoulam's sample are in an alterated position or the inlet-system of the mass spectrometer was not suitable for this kind of product.

Tetrahydrocannabinol III

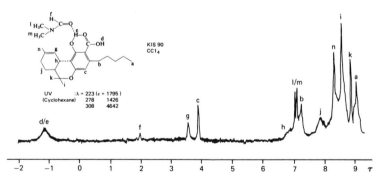

The above compound decomposes on heating while cannabinol and cannabidiol are formed. It is easily cleaved hydrogenolytically giving cannabidiolic acid and a diol. This cleavage is a typical reaction of α-benzylic esters. The position of the OH— groups has not been established exactly. We only know that there are two, one of which must be tertiary. This is the first known compound of this phenolic series which contains two phenolic units. We now know that these compounds obtained from hashish samples are certainly not double bond isomers. These studies have thus shown that only one tetrahydro-cannabinol compound with trans-linked rings and the double bond in the 9,10-position is to be found in considerable amounts.

Fig. 8. NMR spectrum of tetrahydrocannabinol carboxylic acid.

By counter-current distribution we isolated still another product, the tetrahydrocannabinol carboxylic acid (Fig. 8). The formula looks rather complicated; we have isolated this compound as a fairly stable complex with dimethylformamide. The compound has probably been overlooked up to now, because it is not completely stable. We were rather lucky to find it, because in counter-current distribution we use a system containing dimethylformamide. Attempts to decarboxylate this acid to tetrahydrocannabinol have shown that very pure Δ^9-tetrahydrocannabinol can be obtained by this method.

We succeeded in isolating a crystalline product from the tetrahydrocannabinol-fraction and we believed that this was the first proven instance of crystalline tetrahydrocannabinol. But further investigations showed it to have the following structure:

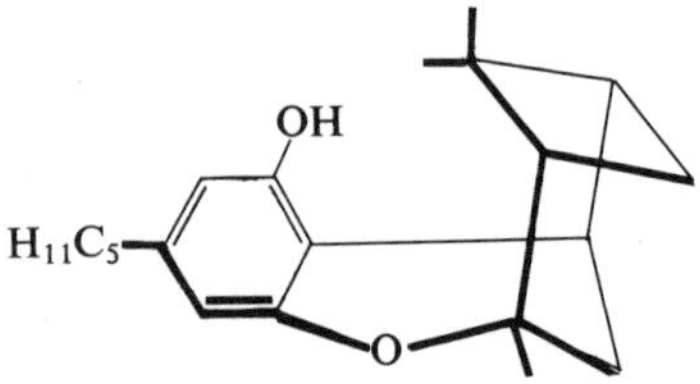

The structure we proposed for cannabipinol (cannabicyclol) on the basis of NMR and MS could not be proved by synthesis. Crombie and Ponsford obtained small amounts of cannabicyclol after condensation of olivetol with citral in the presence of pyridine. Based on this synthesis they proposed a new structure, for which the photochemical cyclization of cannabichromene to cannabicyclol gave further evidence:

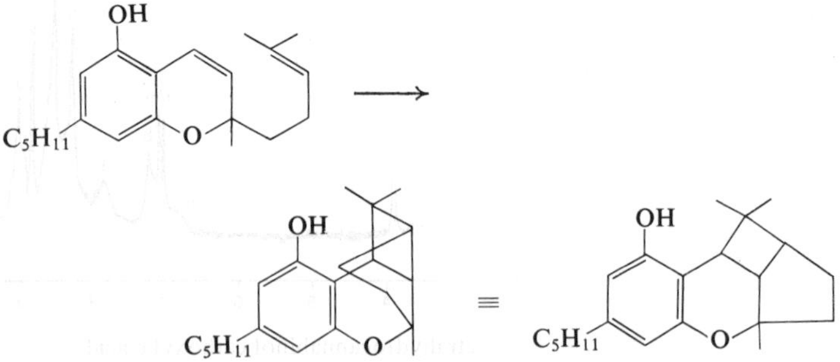

At the end of last year we succeeded in isolating a homologue of cannabidiol, which we called cannabidivarin (CBDV). Cannabidivarin is the first compound found in hashish which has the divarinyl-group (n-propyl-) instead of the usual olivetyl-group. The absolute configuration according to ORD is identical with that of cannabidiol. CBDV synthesized from divarine and *trans*-p-menthadiene-(2,8)-ol-(1) in the presence of N,N-dimethyl-formamide-dimethylacetate is identical in its analytical and spectroscopic data with CBDV isolated from hashish:

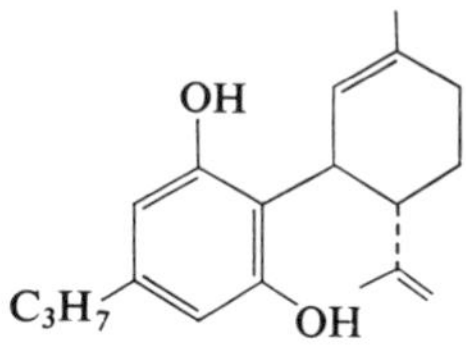

SYNTHESES OF SOME CONSTITUENTS

We were the first to synthesize the CBD-skeleton. We started from olivetol dimethyl ether with lithium and introduced the formyl group. The product was reacted with acetone to yield the benzalacetone, followed by a Diels-Alder reaction with isoprene. This reaction can lead to a product having the acetyl group either in 6- or 5- position. In accordance with the results obtained with similar systems, our experiments showed that the product having the acetyl group in 6-position is formed almost exclusively. The C=O-group could be transferred to the CCH_2-group by a Wittig reaction, giving the CBD-dimethylester. This ether cleavage is rather difficult to carry out in an acidic medium, because there are many by-products, among them tetrahydrocannabinol. For a comparison of natural and synthetic cannabidiol it seemed more convenient to compare their dimethyl ethers, because these are easier to handle. Cannabidiol isolated from the plant was therefore methylated to cannabidiol dimethyl ether. From the fact that the two ethers are different, we concluded that in natural cannabidiol the double bond must be in the 2,3-position. After these studies had been completed, Mechoulam and his colleagues, using the new Varian A-60-NMR equipment, were able to propose the 2,3-position for the double bond and to exclude

Synthesis of cannabidiol (1)

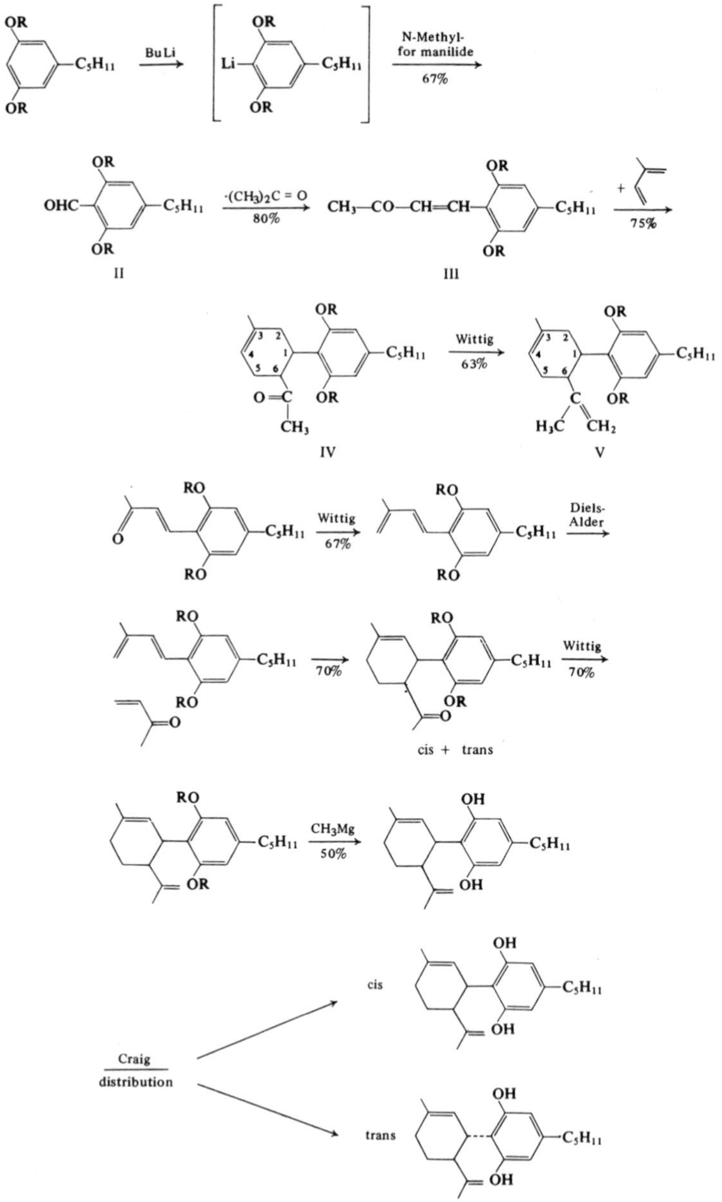

Fig. 9. Synthesis of Cannabidiol.

the 3,4-position. Thus both of us had found by completely indepen-
dent methods that in cannabidiol the double bond must have the
2,3- and not any other position (see Fig. 9).

Then we tried to synthesize cannabidiol, which we considered
likely to be a key structural compound of hashish. This time we
slightly modified the method described before and immediately
carried out the Wittig reaction with the benzalacetone compound, in
order to introduce the isoprene configuration into the molecule.
Subsequently we carried out the Diels-Alder reaction with methyl-
vinylketone to obtain the double bond and then again subjected the
product to a Wittig reaction. Now the ether could be cleaved with
methyl magnesium iodide to the corresponding cannabidiol in a
smooth reaction. Meanwhile, Mechoulam and Gaoni have published
the cyclization of cannabigerol in an acidic medium.

When this cannabidiol is subjected to Craig-, or better, Jantzen-
distribution, it can be partitioned into *cis*- and *trans*-cannabidiol. It
can be shown that synthetic *trans*-cannabidiol and natural cannabidiol
have completely identical properties.

We adhered to this note of synthesis only changing the ether groups,
because it is fairly difficult to cleave the dimethylether. Many groups
were tried; the dihydropyran gave the most satisfactory results. When
carrying out this reaction with the pyran group, the homologue of
tetrahydrocannabinol is obtained without great difficulty.

Summing up, we can say that a large number of compounds are

known which are all somehow structurally related to tetrahydro-cannabinol. They are open-chained compounds, dehydration products or something of the kind. The only compounds occurring in plants are cannabidiol carboxylic acid and *trans*-tetrahydrocannabinol acid. It has been proved that cannabidiol is formed from this cannabidiol carboxylic acid and that tetrahydrocannabinol can be obtained from this cannabidiol by chemical reaction.

Of the compounds isolated by us, tetrahydrocannabinol was the only one to show any notable psychomimetric activity in the tests upon human beings carried out at Lexington. We have isolated the tetrahydrocannabinol carboxylic acid under the assumption that it is the unstable precursor of tetrahydrocannabinol, the active hashish principle. However, we have not been able to furnish any evidence for this assumption, because a variety of compounds was obtained, the constitution of which has not yet been determined.

The above formula illustrates those structural elements which ought to be responsible for the hashish activity on the basis of the test results obtained by Dr. Isbell in Lexington. The stereo model of tetrahydro-cannabinol shows that there is a gap in the cyclohexene ring which is caused by the trans-linkage. Dimethylformamide or similar compounds could well fit into this gap, which also accounts for the formation of a 1:1 complex of the tetrahydrocannabinol carboxylic acid. We postulate that this gap and this tendency of tetrahydrocannabinol to form a complex is of importance regarding the point of attack in the brain and is responsible for the physiological activity.

SUMMARY

Δ^9-Tetrahydrocannabinol (THC) is the only compound isolated from hashish which has so far shown hashish activity, while all other compounds so far isolated are inactive. THC is an artificial product not to be found in fresh plant material; this also applies to cannabidiol.

Today it is relatively easy to synthesize all the known tetrahydro-cannabinols, except the naturally occurring tetrahydrocannabinol isomer. It appears that we have now reached the stage where routes of synthesis are available that can enable us to modify considerably the structure of the THC molecule, to discover its point of attack in the brain, and to find out to what extent this varies when different hetero atoms are introduced into the molecule. In our opinion, all chemical problems about hashish have been solved and only pharmacological problems remain.

References

Claussen, U., Borger, W. and Korte, F., *Liebigs Ann. Chem.* 693:165 (1966).

Claussen, U., Fehlhaber, H. W. and Korte, F., *Tetrahedron*, 22:3535 (1966).

Claussen, U. and Korte, F., *Tetrahedron, Suppl. No.* 7:89 (1965).

Claussen, U. and Korte, F., *Z. Naturfschg.* 21b:594 (1966a).

Claussen, U. and Korte, F., *Die Naturwissenschaften*, 21:541 (1966b).

Claussen, U. and Korte, F., *Tetrahedron*, 24:5379 (1968a).

Claussen, U. and Korte, F., *Liebigs Ann. Chem.* 713:162 (1968b).

Claussen, U., Mummenhoff, P. and Korte, F., *Tetrahedron,* 24:2897 (1968).

Claussen, U., Spulak, F. v. and Korte, F., *Tetrahedron,* 22:1477 (1966).

Claussen, U., Spulak, F. v. and Korte, F., *Tetrahedron,* 24:1021 (1968).

Crombie, L. and Ponsford, R., *Tetrahedron Letters,* 55:5771 (1968).

Isbell, H., Gorodetzsky, C. W., Jasinski, D., Claussen, U., Spulak, F. V. and Korte, F., *Psychopharmacologia* (Berl) 11:184 (1967).

Korte, F. and Bieniek, D., *Materia Medica Nordmark* XX/11:607 (1968).

Korte, F., Dlugosch, E. and Claussen, U., *Liebigs Ann. Chem.* 693:165 (1966).

Korte, F., Haag, M. and Claussen, U., *Angew. Chem.* 77:862 (1965).

Korte, F. and Sieper, H., *Liebigs Ann. Chem.* 630:71 (1960a).

Korte, F. and Sieper, H., *Tetrahedron,* 10:153 (1960b).

Korte, F. and Sieper, H., *J. Chromatog.* 13:90 (1964a).

Korte, F. and Sieper, H., *J. Chromatog.* 14:178 (1964b).

Vollner, L., Bieniek, D. and Korte, F., *Tetrahedron Letters,* 3:145 (1969).

4 Studies on Cannabis Constituents and Synthetic Analogues

R. K. Razdan and H. G. Pars

It has been generally accepted that the active constituents of *Cannabis indica* are I and II, i.e., Δ^1-3,4-*trans*-tetrahydrocannabinol (THC), and Δ^6-3,4-*trans*-THC respectively (Mechoulam and Gaoni, 1967).

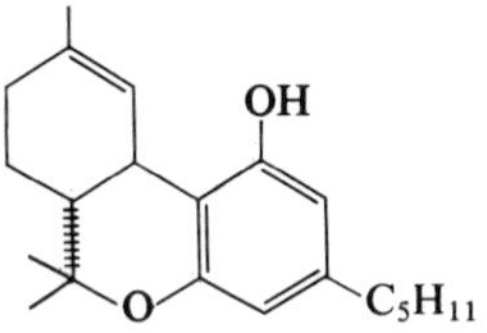

I

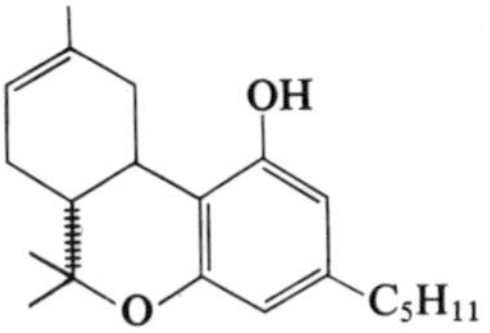

II

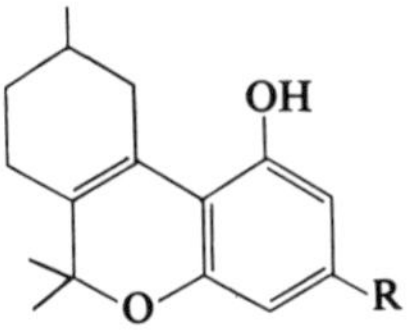

III

During the study of natural cannabinoids synthetic compounds based on formula III were prepared by Adams. Adams showed that the degree of activity in these compounds varied with the alkyl substituent R, the most potent compound being the dimethylheptyl derivative (R = CH—CH–(CH$_2$)$_4$–CH$_3$). This was found, in dog-ataxia studies, to be approximately 500 times more active than the compound in which R = C$_5$H$_{11}$ (Adams, Harfenist and Loewe, 1949).

NITROGEN ANALOGUES

It was considered of interest to synthesize the aza or alkaloidal analogues of THC since, besides THC, there are few agents known to be active in the CNS, but containing no nitrogen. Therefore, in designing such nitrogen analogues, the following factors were considered: (a) phenethylamine orientation as found in the large majority of aromatic alkaloids (e.g. phenethylamines, morphine, indoles, indolylethylamines; (b) aryl tetrahydropyridine moiety, which is found in particular in psychotomimetic agents (e.g. LSD, yohimbine); and (c) aryl piperidine moiety, which is present in many agents active upon the CNS. Furthermore, we find some additional points of similarity in the structures of morphine, THC and LSD:

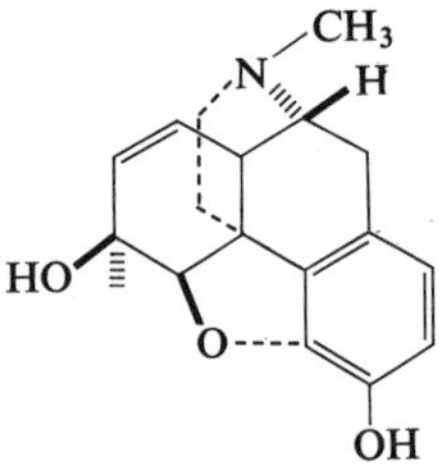

Morphine 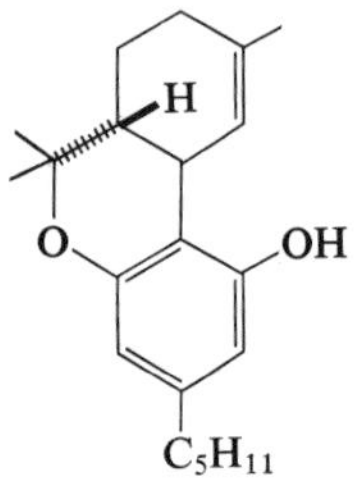 Δ^1-THC

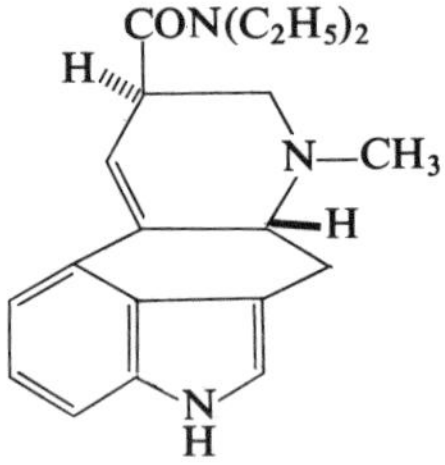

LSD

All have a planar ring (benzene in the case of morphine and Δ^1-THC, and indole in LSD) joined to a β-hydrogen atom two carbon atoms away.

Keeping in view the above considerations, the nitrogen analogue IV and its dihydro derivatives were synthesized. Interestingly, they are active on the CNS, and produce ataxia and motor deficits in mice, cats, dogs, and monkeys (Pars, Granchelli, Keller and Razdan, 1966).

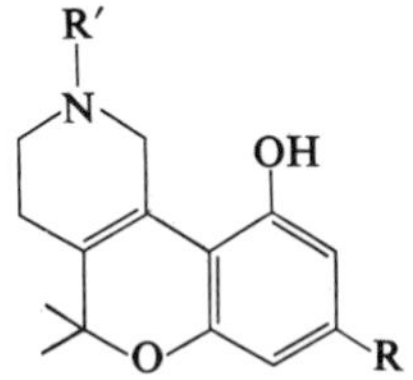

IV (3,4-d-aza THC) 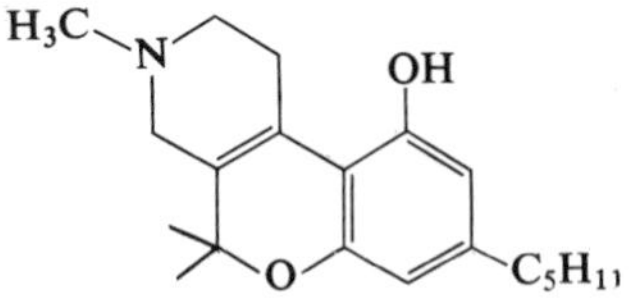   V (3,4-c-aza THC)

This is not surprising if one considers the striking structural similarity between the nitrogen analogue IV and LSD, and another nitrogen analogue V and morphine, as shown below:

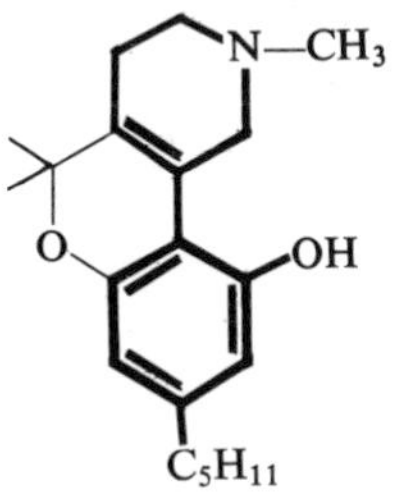

IV 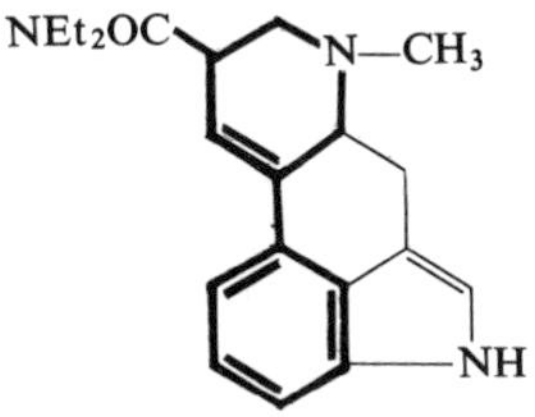   LSD

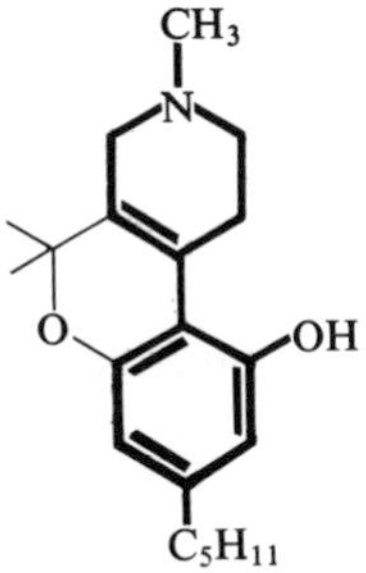

V 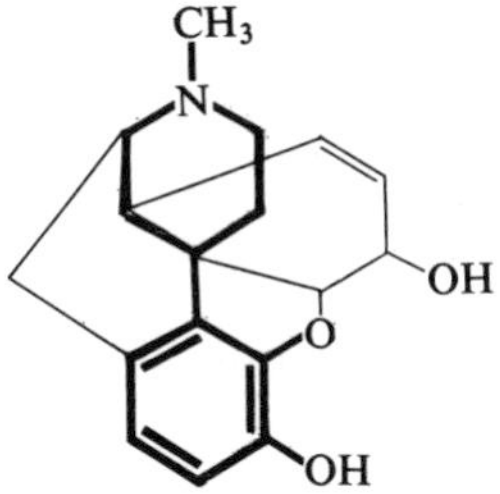   Morphine

It is interesting that Ankar and Cook (1946) (see also Barlow, 1955) synthesized compound V and its dihydro derivative in 1946 and reported it to have no analgesic activity. No mention was made of other CNS activity of these compounds.

Further classes of THC analogues which we have synthesized are the following (Razdan, Thompson, Pars and Granchelli, 1967; Razdan,

Pars, Granchelli and Harris, 1968; and Pars, Granchelli, Keller, Razdan, Van Horn, Hunneman, Shoer, Thompson, Harris and Dewey, 1967):

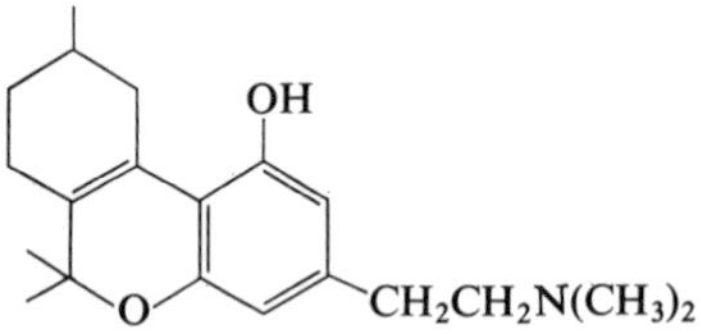

VI

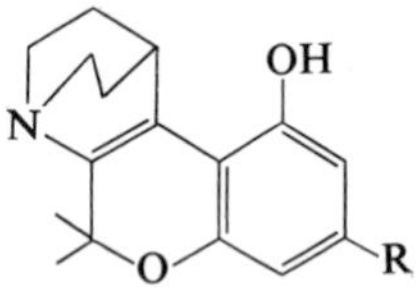

3,4-b-aza THC
VII

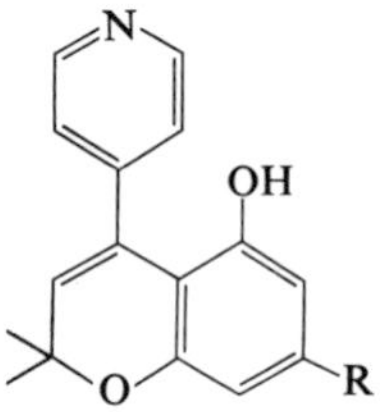

VIII

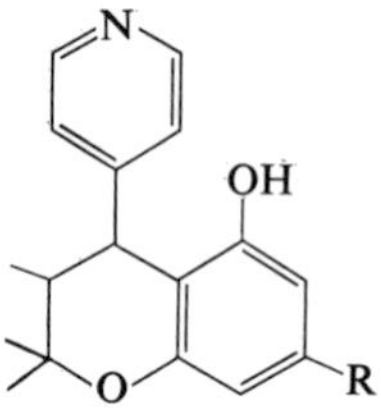

IX

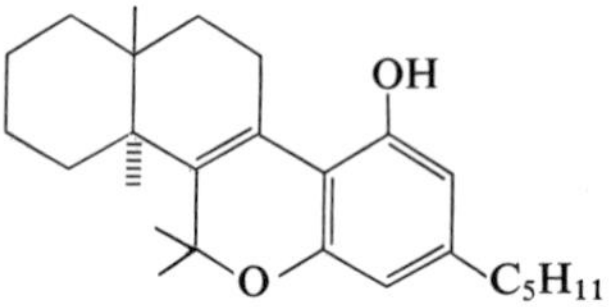

X

They are all active on the CNS except the steroidal analogue (X).

CANNABIS CONSTITUENTS AND OTHER ANALOGUES

We have recently reported a one-step total synthesis of *dl*-cannabicyclol and *dl*-cannabichromene, the two minor constituents of hashish (Kane and Razdan, 1968 and 1969). This has been achieved by heating an equimolar mixture of citral, olivetol and pyridine. In addition, the tetracyclic ether (XII) is obtained from this reaction mixture, which is converted to iso-THC (XIII) on acid treatment. This is a general reaction and by using this procedure one can synthesize substituted tetracyclic ethers, chromenes and iso-THC. Similar results have been obtained by Crombie and Ponsford (1968).

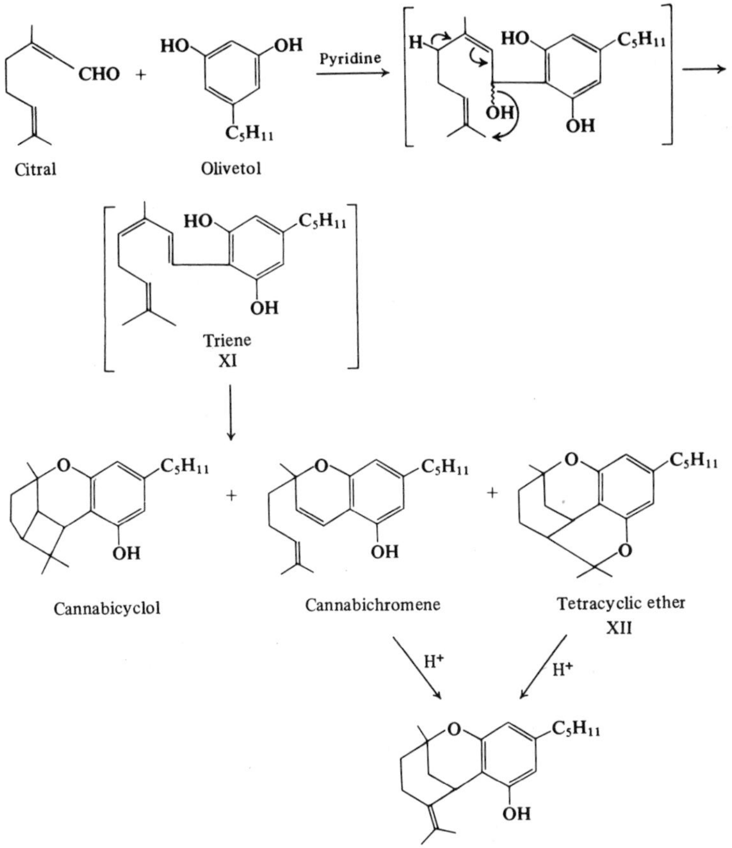

Scheme.

From this reaction mixture we have now isolated an additional compound, for which we propose structure XIV, possessing a four-membered cyclic peroxide ring.

Recently Kopecky and Mumford (1969) have reported the synthesis of 3,3,4-trimethyl-1,2-dioxetane (XV). This is the first example of isolation of a dioxetane, although the products from a number of reactions have been explained as occurring via such four-membered

XIV
(Figures are NMR data)

XV
(Figures are NMR data)

cyclic peroxides (Swern, Coleman and Knight, 1953; Aurich, 1964; Huber, 1968).

We have found that further extraction of the reaction mixture discussed above, with 12:88 and 15:85 ether-petroleum ether (B.P. 30-40°), gave a yellowish oil. This was re-chromatographed on thick silica gel plates to give a colourless resin in 5% yield, homogeneous on thin-layer chromatography. Other data: NMR (CDCl$_3$), δ 0.84 (3H, t, ω-CH$_3$), 1.18, 1.28 (6H, 2s), 1.52 (3H, s), 2.12 (1H, double doublet, J = 3 and 14 cps), 3.44 (1H, m, J = 6 and 14 cps), 4.95 (1H, d, J = 3 cps), 6.34 (1H, d, J = 3 cps aromatic H), 6.41 (1H, d, J = 3 cps, aromatic H), 6.2 (1H, broad, OH; D$_2$O exchangeable); λ_{max}^{EtOH} 280 (ε2170) and 222 mμ sh (ε8670); ir (cm^{-1}, CCl$_4$) 3610 (OH), 1330 (s, ether), 895 (m) and 850 (w) (0-0 stretching). The mass spectrum indicates a molecular ion peak m/e 346 corresponding to C$_{21}$H$_{30}$O$_4$. The compound gives a positive peroxide test.

The presence of only one exchangeable proton in the nmr and the absence of infra-red absorption band in the 3560 cm^{-1} (non-bonded, typical of hydroperoxides) region rules out the presence of a hydroperoxide structure. The position of the C-1 methyl singlet at 1.52 ppm and the C-6 proton at 4.95 ppm is in excellent agreement with the dioxetane XV. Furthermore, on the basis of double resonance experiments (100 Mc/s) the multiplet at δ2.12 is assigned to one of the C-5 protons. The irradiation experiments also indicate a small, long-range coupling between the C-3 benzylic proton (δ3.44) and the C-5 proton at δ2.12.

We were unable to determine the coupling constant for the C-3/C-4 interaction. However, since in Δ^1-3,4-*cis*-tetrahydrocannabinol the benzylic C-3 proton is more de-shielded by the aromatic ring than in the *trans*-isomer (Mechoulam and Gaoni, 1967), the position of benzylic C-3 proton in compound XIV indicates a *cis*-stereochemistry at the ring fusion.

When compound XIV was passed through a gas chromatography column (10% SE-31 on 80-100 mesh chromosorb W; gas helium; oven temperature, 220°), a single peak was observed. Its mass spectrum showed a molecular ion peak m/e 314 (different from XIV i.e. less 32) and in addition included peaks at 299 (M^+-CH_3), 271 ($M^+-C_3H_7$), 258 ($M^+-C_4H_8$), 246, 231 (base) and 193, which are characteristic of tetrahydrocannabinols (Budzikiewicz, Alpin, Lightner, Djerassi, Mechoulam and Gaoni, 1965; Claussen, Fehlhaber and Korte, 1966).

Catalytic hydrogenation of compound XIV in the presence of 10% palladium/charcoal in methanol for 16 hr afforded a crystalline compound, mp 94-95° to which we assign structure XVI. Data: NMR $CDCl_3$), δ0.88 (3H, t, ω-CH_3), 1.11, 1.25 (6H, 2s, gem dimethyl), 1.41 (3H, s), 2.5 (1H, m), 3.55 (3H, s, $-OCH_3$), 4.84 (1H, d, J = 7 cps, hemiacetal), 4.0, 5.94 (2H, broad, D_2O exchangeable), 6.18 (1H, d, J = 3 cps aromatic H), 6.31 (1H, d, J = 3 cps, aromatic H); ir (cm^{-1}, KBr) 3430, 3200 (OH) and 1190 (m), 1130 (s), 1075 (m), 1035 (m); (C–O–C–O–C bands). The mass spectrum confirmed the molecular composition $C_{22}H_{34}O_5$, and in addition included peaks at 360 (M^+-H_2O), 346 (M^+-CH_3OH), 331 and 288 (base) which are completely explicable on the basis of structure XVI. The methyl singlet at 1.41 ppm and the hemiacetal proton at 4.84 ppm are in agreement with literature values in similar compounds (Dolby, Ellinger, Esfandiori and Marshall, 1968; Bhacca, Johnson and Shoolery, 1962). Similarly, the slight shift in the position of gem dimethyl groups in XVI is in accordance with that reported by Gaoni and Mechoulam (1968) in the case of l-methoxy-hexahydrocannabinol. Compound XVI gives a positive test with Tollens reagent. This is taken as confirmation of the presence of hemiacetal function. Moreover, it furnished a resinous 2,4-dinitrophenylhydrazone of the acid (XVII) ($C_{27}H_{34}N_2O_8$:m/e 542) which was purified by chromatography on thick silica gel plates. Oxidative properties of 2,4-dinitrophenylhydrazone are known (Welti and Whittaker, 1962).

XVI

XVII

We suggest that the most reasonable interpretation of the mechanisms of formation of compound XVI is the following:

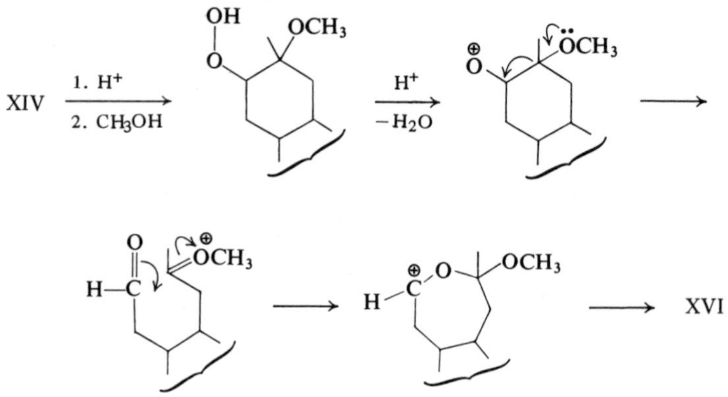

Similar rearrangements of hydroperoxides are known (Hawkins, 1961). In confirmation of this proposed scheme, compound XVI was also formed when compound XIV was treated with a catalytic amount of p-toluenesulphonic acid in methanol for 16 hr.

PHARMACOLOGICAL RESULTS

Preliminary results from these compounds have been presented previously (Razdan, Kane, Pars, Kucera, Reid, Harris, Dewey and Howes, 1968); results are given in Tables I and II. The primary screen data (Table I) was determined by modified Irwin technique (Irwin, 1964). The data presented in Table II was determined at 50 mg/kg (i.v.) and 100 mg/kg (p.o.) dose level. For analgesic studies we utilized the tail-flick procedure (Harris and Pierson, 1964) and the anti-writhing test in mice (Pearl and Harris, 1966). The prevention and reversal of reserpine-induced ptosis in mice was investigated with the method of Aceto and Harris (1965). Cardiovascular and respiratory studies were carried out in anaesthetized dogs (sodium thiopentone, 15 mg/kg, followed by sodium barbitone, 225 mg/kg i.v.) using essentially the same technique as described by Harris (1964).

TABLE 1.

Compound	Dose mg/kg	Route	Effect
Δ^9-THC	10.0	i.v. s.c.	Very aggressive and vocal when touched; otherwise depressed.
Δ^8-THC	10.0	i.v. s.c.	Very aggressive, piloerection, performance on vertical rod very difficult; otherwise depressed.
Cannabichromene	10.0 15-30	s.c. s.c.	Passive, slight loss of neuromuscular coordination. Cyanosis, urination increased.
Cannabicyclol	10.0	i.v. (PEG 200)	Irritable when touched; piloerection, flushed, increased respiration.
iso-THC	10.0	i.v.	Aggressive, increased reactivity.
Tetracyclic Ether	100.0	i.v. (PEG 200)	Suggestion of depression

TABLE 2.

Compound	Tail Flick IV	Tail Flick PO	Writhing IV	Writhing PO	Inc. Screen IV	Inc. Screen PO	Roto Rod IV	Roto Rod PO	Reserpine Reversal IV	Reserpine Reversal PO	Reserpine Prevention IV	Reserpine Prevention PO
Δ^9-THC	1.4%	1.2	76	68	0/12	0/11	1/12	1/11	0	0	5%	–
Δ^8-THC	7.1%	14.6	0	33	0/12	0/11	0/12	1/11	2.5%	18%	20%	–
Cannabicyclol	0	–	0	–	0/12	–	0/12	–	0	–	–	–
Cyclic Ether	0	–	22	–	0/12	–	0/12	–	0	–	–	–

DISCUSSION

These results indicate that Δ^9-THC may have more analgesic activity than Δ^8-THC, whereas the latter may have more stimulatory activity as evidenced by the prevention and reversal of ptosis induced by reserpine in mice. In our opinion the most significant result is the catecholamine potentiation by both Δ^1- and Δ^6-THC derivatives. All effects of noradrenaline and adrenaline are potentiated as shown in Figs. 1 and 2. This might account for the euphoric effects associated with marihuana.

Acknowledgements   The helpful collaboration of L. S. Harris, V. V. Kane, and F. E. Granchelli for their contribution to this paper is gratefully acknowledged. We thank K. A. Kopecky and C. Mumford for spectral data on compound XV.

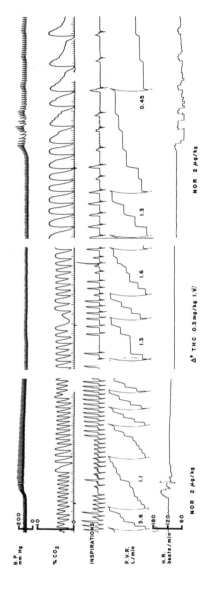

Fig. 1. Effect of noradrenaline (NOR) and Δ⁹-THC on various measures of physiological activity.

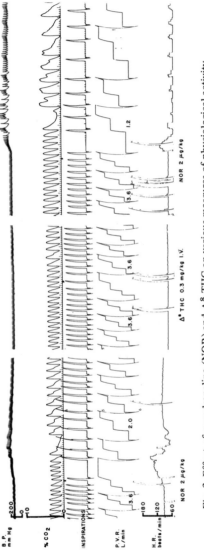

Fig. 2. Effect of noradrenaline (NOR) and Δ⁸-THC on various measures of physiological activity.

References

Aceto, M. D. and Harris, L. S., *Toxicol. Appl. Pharmacol.* 7:329 (1965)

Adams, R., Harfenist, M. and Loewe, S., *J. Am. Chem. Soc.* 71:1624 (1949).

Anker, R. M. and Cook, A. H., *J. Chem. Soc.* 58 (1946).

Aurich, H. G., *Tetrahedron Letters,* 657 (1964).

Barlow, R. B., "Introduction to Chemical Pharmacology", p. 47, Methuen and Co., Ltd., London (1955).

Bhacca, N. S., Johnson, L. F. and Shoolery, J. N., "High Resolution NMR Spectra Catalogue", Vol. 1:143, Varian Assoc., U.S.A. (1962).

Budzikiewicz, H., Alpin, R. T., Lightner, D. A., Djerassi, C., Mechoulam, R. and Gaoni, Y., *Tetrahedron,* 21:1881 (1965).

Claussen, U., Fehlhaber, H. W. and Korte, F., *Tetrahedron,* 22:3535 (1966).

Crombie, L. and Ponsford, R., *Chem. Commun.* 894 (1968); *Tetrahedron Letters,* 4557 (1968).

Dolby, L. J., Elliger, C. A., Esfandiori, S. and Marshall, K. S., *J. Org. Chem.* 33:4508 (1968).

Gaoni, Y. and Mechoulam, R., *Israel J. Chem.* 6:679 (1968).

Harris, L. S., *Arch. Exp. Pathol. Pharmak.* 248:426 (1964).

Harris, L. S. and Pierson, A. K., *J. Pharmacol.* 143:144 (1964).

Hubner, J. E., *Tetrahedron Letters,* 3271 (1968).

Hawkins, E. G. E., "Organic Peroxides", p. 54, D. Van Nostrand Co., Inc., Princeton, N.J., (1961).

Irwin, S., "Pharmacologic Techniques in Drug Evaluation" (Chapter 4), Nadine, J. H. and Siegler, P. E., eds., Year Book Medical Publishers, Inc., Chicago (1964).

Kane, V. V. and Razdan, R. K., *J. Am. Chem. Soc.* 90:6551 (1968), *Tetrahedron Letters,* 591 (1969).

Kopecky, K. R. and Mumford, C., *Canad. J. Chem.* 47:709 (1969).

Mechoulam, R. and Gaoni, Y., *Fortschr. Chem. Org. Naturstoffe,* 25:175 (1967).

Pars, H. G., Granchelli, F. E., Keller, J. K. and Razdan, R. K., *J. Am. Chem. Soc.,* 88:3664 (1966).

Pars, H. G., Granchelli, F. E., Keller, J. K., Razdan, R. K., Shoer, L., Thompson, W. R., Harris, L. S. and Dewey, W. L., *Chimica Therapeutica,* 2:167 (1967).

Pars, H. G., Granchelli, F. E., Keller, J. K., Razdan, R. K., Van Horn, S. and Hunneman, D., 1st Int. Cong. Hetr. Chem. Albuquerque, N. Mexico, June 1967.

Pearl, J. and Harris, L. S., *J. Pharmacol. Expt. Ther.* 154:319 (1966).

Razdan, R. K., Kane, V. V., Pars, H. G., Kucera, J. L., Reid, D. H., Harris, L. S. Dewey, W. L. and Howes, J. F., Minutes, 30th Meeting, Committee on Problems of Drug Dependence, NAS-NRC, (1968) in press.

Razdan, R. K., Thompson, W. R., Pars, H. G. and Granchelli, F. E., *Tetrahedron Letters,* 3405 (1967).

Razdan, R. K., Pars, H. G., Granchelli, F. E. and Harris, L. S., *J. Med. Chem.* 11:377 (1968).

Swern, D., Coleman, J. E. and Knight, H. B., *J. Am. Chem. Soc.* 75:3135 (1953).

Welti, D. and Whittaker, D., *Chem. Ind.* 986 (1962).

DISCUSSION 2: CHEMICAL AND PHYSICOCHEMICAL ASPECTS

(a) Solubility; Extraction of cannabinoids from plant material; stability of acidic materials.

Fairbairn   Aqueous sodium hydroxide does not normally dissolve THC. Alcoholic caustic soda is generally used.

Mechoulam   A petroleum ether extract of plant material has most of the cannabinoids in it. Then one can extract most of the acidic cannabinoids from it with aqueous sodium hydroxide.

Fairbairn   But not the non-acidic compounds?

Mechoulam   No, definitely not, although these are phenolic: this is one thing that has always puzzled people. They are not really acidic, in the sense that frequently the free phenols will not dissolve in basic solution; only the carboxylic acids will do this, and even these do not always do so. THC acid dissolves only moderately.

Razdan   The partition of other isomers with even longer side-chains is completely changed.

Fairbairn   Professor Krejci, do you drop the plant straight into alcohol, immediately after collection and drying?

Krejci   Yes.

Fairbairn   At this stage you have the acidic form and not the decarboxylated form? The fresh plant contains the carboxylated form, and on drying loses the carboxyl group, to give THC and cannabidiol itself. Does this happen on drying?

Korte   If you chromatograph the petroleum ether extract of the intact plant you find all the phenolic compounds, as well as the carboxylic acid, but you also find tetrahydrocannabinol, cannabidiol and so on. In fluid from the fresh-growing plant, we could only find cannabidiol, and the carboxylic acid. After drying and storing at $0°C$ you find cannabidiol.

Mechoulam   Dr. Schultes said that cannabis is notorious for its cultivars and chemovars, so I do not see any difficulty in concluding that in some countries there are types of cannabis which do not decarboxylate. We do not know why this would occur, maybe the process is enzymatic, maybe not. This is the only conclusion we can come to about differences in the results from Greece and other countries.

Fairbairn   Decarboxylation would not happen spontaneously: it would have to be enzymatic, would it not?

Mechoulam   Not necessarily, no.

Fairbairn   What sort of temperature would be needed?

Mechoulam For laboratory decarboxylation, about 103°C, but I think it is a question of kinetics. Perhaps it may decarboxylate spontaneously or on standing for a long time.

Paton Trace elements may be relevant again here.

Shulgin You may have a catalytic decarboxylation, with differences between one area and another due to regional differences in trace ions. This would not be an enzymatic phenomenon.

Braenden The United Nations Laboratory has arranged for the experimental cultivation under different ecological conditions of cannabis seeds from the same batches. These seeds (from cannabis grown in Lebanon, South Africa and Switzerland) were grown in countries ranging from Senegal to Norway and, so far, material from this ecological study has been received from Norway, Spain and Switzerland. Similar experiments were carried out earlier with the same batches of seeds in Denmark and the Federal Republic of Germany. In 1968 cannabis was successfully grown even in very far northern latitudes. The results from this study may be relevant to the point.

(b) Potency of substances given by mouth or by inhalation

Fairbairn If 98% decomposes during smoking, only two per cent reaches the lung?

Korte Yes, under the conditions that we used. If you change the smoking conditions, I am sure you will get other results.

Fairbairn How did you give it orally—THC is not very soluble in water.

Korte In olive oil.

Fairbairn That means that it seems to be 250 times as powerful when smoked as when taken orally, because only 2% of the smoked material reaches the lung.

Joyce We do not know how much of it, given by either route, actually reaches the effective sites; so this is a rather unreal kind of ratio and inferences from it must be cautious.

Korte This ratio corresponds with the practical experience of the users of hashish, who prefer inhalation to an oral dose.

Razdan Either it is as potent as you say, or the active principle is, at least in part, due to something else. The Japanese have also pointed out that Indian charas had very little Δ^1, whereas the Japanese variety had a lot more: yet it is known to be much less effective. So there is another conflict of opinions.

Mechoulam There is no conflict here. Professor Isbell used pure THC, not a mixture, and found activity on a weight basis at the level of LSD.

Bein   If 98% is burned, the activity does not matter. Under Professor
Korte's conditions, 98% is combusted. Nobody in this room knows
whether this holds true for Isbell's experiments. For instance, the
rate of smoking might influence the data.

Miras   I would like to say that in our somewhat similar experiment,
only 40% was lost in the smoking machine. We used a radioactive
method. THC was still present after smoking, as well as cannabidiol;
cannabidiolic acid disappeared. Also, smoking is distillation in vacuum,
and the technique with which hashish users smoke the cigarette is
probably important, as well as the way in which they make it.

Korte   It is also difficult to collect the smoke which comes from
the machine and to condense it completely.

Lister   In your joint paper with Dr. Isbell, did you not suggest that
the effects produced implied that there was another active component?

Korte   Yes. 70% can be related to the THC concentration, but no
other isolated phenol shows any activity. On the other hand, we do
not know anything about synergistic activity between possible
components.

Mechoulam   In your observation that only 70% of the activity of
crude material is present in the pure material, what was the basis for
assay of the former—THC, or THC plus THC acids?

Korte   The TCH concentration in hashish.

Mechoulam   How was that measured?

Korte   Chemically. We gave Dr. Isbell several samples containing a
normal concentration of THC. He compared them all with standardized, pure THC.

Mechoulam   Both tetrahydrocannabinolic acids decarboxylate on
smoking, so they are essentially active material and one must take
this into account in the analysis. I wonder if by the time the material
is transported from one place to the other, some of it is destroyed.

Korte   We have checked this; there is no evidence for decomposition.

Mechoulam   Does the loss of 30% make a significant difference?

Korte   According to Isbell's experience and that of the subjects, yes.

Paton   If "70% effective" means that the relative maximum effect
achievable falls short by 30%, and that this is not something that can
be remedied by increasing the dose, I should have thought that it
could not merely be due to the THC concentration.

Mechoulam   I do not think that Isbell has published any such 70%
figure. We should wait for such a publication before speculating
further.

(c) Effect of substitutents on activity

Mechoulam   We have to see Adams' results, which Dr. Razdan quoted,

*in perspective; dog ataxia is not really anything that can be compared
with the results of human testing.*

Razdan   We feel exactly the same. This is merely the background.

Mechoulam   We have tested our derivatives with side-chains, as
Adams did, and we have found a little potentiation, for example with
a dimethyl-7 side-chain: which, however, according to some reports,
is 500 times as potent.

Razdan   This dimethyl-7 side-chain is really magical. We are trying
to investigate what is so magical about it.

Mechoulam   We did not find so great an increase in monkeys.

Razdan   The ratio may be quite different in monkeys from that in
dog ataxia because the dog is especially susceptible in this test; as in
the case of vomiting.

Mechoulam   I think that the dog is not a very good animal for the
purpose. In the 1,6 compounds with a dimethylheptyl side-chain, we
have found up to 10 times more activity, but not 500 times more.
The Δ^1 compound may give a better result; we have not done much
with it yet. It is, however, a very potent compound, with long-term
activity instead of a couple of hours; in the monkey it acts for about
three days—a very interesting compound. Isbell also tested the isomer
and another major compound; the synthetic compound on which
Adams based his results. Professor Korte has prepared it again and
given it to Isbell who finds that it is not active in humans in the doses
in which he tested it.

Korte   That is correct.

Mechoulam   This is very surprising, because the compound was
actually on the market with a C-6 side-chain, as Synhexyl. If indeed
it is not active, a very thorough re-examination must be made of this
whole series of compounds.

Paton   Is it possible that what was on the market was in fact an
impure substance?

Mechoulam   Yes, it is possible.

Korte   In animals Synhexyl is active.

Bein   It is said that the human activity of the compound which was
on the American market was always very doubtful.

Paton   The old animal work is extremely difficult to interpret. The
corneal anaesthesia test is very difficult to perform. If you find areas
of disagreement with a factor of 10, I am not surprised. I think I would
worry much more if somebody said it was totally inactive.

Mechoulam   This was supposed to be totally inactive in humans,
which is very surprising.

Joyce   The original clinical tests of Synhexyl were made in the days before controlled trials. Whatever the appropriate control might be—a placebo or some other kind of active control substance—the answer should be much clearer with an appropriately designed clinical trial under modern conditions.

Shulgin   Does the $\Delta^{1,6}$ compound have a 9-carbon chain? A third and a fourth isomeric centre would again double the isomers. This might possibly be the reason for the difference, the fivefold increase in yours, as opposed to Adams', compound. Was there any stereo-isomeric centre in your compound?

Mechoulam   We did not think it worthwhile to separate the isomers. We thought that we would be getting more or less equal amounts of every isomer. Most probably we and Adams got the same kind of mixture of all the compounds, within a reasonable range.

(d) Structure-activity

Lister   I would like to ask Professor Petrzilka to elaborate on the effects of his chlorocompound. He said it showed tranquillizing properties. Were those properties qualitatively different from those of THC itself? Was it more like chlorpromazine?

Petrzilka   It was similar, yes, without specifying exactly the details of how it was assessed.

Paton   I have always felt that one of the worst vices of the pharmo-cologist is to take unrelated chemical structures and try to force them into similar patterns! Chemists also do just this on occasions. I think one turns to the chemist for a different sort of job. I recall the chemical pharmacologist, Dr. Raymond Ing, saying a long time ago: "People claim that ephedrine and noradrenaline are structurally very alike, and therefore they must have the same pharmacology. In fact, it is obvious that their pharmacology must be different because ephedrine has a significant vapour pressure". And, of course, their pharmacology is different: ephedrine is believed to act largely by mobilizing amines whereas noradrenaline acts directly.

I think I would prefer chemists to talk about "the reactions of which a compound is capable". Then, in ten or a hundred years, when we know the structure of a cell membrane, for example, we may be able to say: "Yes, this compound might react there".

Crombie   Could I make some defence of the chemists, not having indulged in this vice myself? Perhaps the parable of recent advances with the synthetic pyrethrin insecticides is instructive. Here, specu-lations of the kind to which you object were made and did in fact lead to a synthetic insecticide that was many times as active as the natural pyrethrins. Whether the speculation is scientifically correct

or not, it may well initiate further work, and this seems to me the
real scientific justification for it. Let men speculate, let them test
out their hypotheses, and we shall discover new things.

Paton   The pharmaceutical industry needs roughly 5,000 speculations
per new drug! What I am really arguing is that one should sharpen the
speculations.

Fairbairn   Professor Petrzilka did not make any reference to
resemblances to 5-HT.

Paton   I would have thought the structural clues are trivial compared
to the fact that there is good evidence that there are at least three
transmitters in the brain: 5-HT, noradrenaline, and acetyl choline,
and it is sensible to talk about them on biochemical or physiological
grounds. I do not think one needs any other reason, but if one is to
speculate, glycine or something like that is important in the central
nervous system, and one can start speculating about other aminoacids.
Picrotoxin and strychnine can also be mentioned, and many other
substances ought to be brought into this game, if one plays it at all.

(e) Discussion: Scientific and Other Consequences of Synthesis of THC

Fairbairn   It looks as though one could synthesize a number of these
compounds fairly readily. There is already in this country an organization to try and synthesize some of this material. Will the members
of this organization run up against the Dangerous Drugs Act? A second
question is whether there is now much reason to work on the plant.
If the pharmocologists want to work on the active principles, perhaps
they should now just leave it to the chemists; they no longer need to
go to people who grow the plant?

Mechoulam   The official drugs acts are being changed; in Israel they
have been changed. Synthetic THC is now controlled there. In the
United States there is a legal difference between synthetic and natural
THC; there are two different laws, and it is certainly better to work
with synthetic products, because the laws are better.

   I believe that most countries will have to change their laws, since
it is very simple to synthesize crude THC if olivetol is available.

Fairbairn   Where does one get olivetol at the moment?

Mechoulam   Hopefully, nowhere. We synthesize it. Most people
synthesize their own. It is not difficult for an organic plant to do so.
NIMH is getting it made commercially, I believe, but the company
in question will only sell it to governments.

Razdan   Olivetol is now available commercially in the States. It has
been advertised by a company in New Jersey in the newspapers, so
you can really buy it on the open market.

Joyce   Before we can attach too much importance to so-called pure

substances, we must show that the pure substances are identical to
the crude substances, and at present this is not proved.
Fairbairn   Pure synthetic THC will have exactly the same effect as
Professor Korte's extract, will it not?
Joyce   No, this is the point. He found only 70% of the activity
present in the pure material. There is another aspect that should be
considered. The really interesting effects of cannabis upon human
beings may be due to interactions between different components
present in the naturally occurring raw material, but separated by
extraction or by synthesis.
Mechoulam   I believe it is much easier to obtain THC in large quantities from plants by partial synthesis via cannabidiol, which is pure
and convertible into pure THC. With adequate plant and supplies of
raw material, it could be done in kilogram quantities.

(f) Non-cannabinoid constituents of cannabis

Joyce   Everybody seems to have been overlooking, or perhaps skirting,
another problem that is very much in the minds of organic chemists
and botanists. A whole range of other compounds—alkaloids, indoles
in particular, may be present in the cannabis plant. So nothing has
been said about any group of substances except the cannabinols.
Mechoulam   As far as I am aware there are no alkaloids in cannabis.
We have tried to isolate nitrogen-containing compounds without
success, except for some very simple ones. We have not found any
indoles or alkaloids.
Joyce   I have been asked by Professor C. A. Salemink of Utrecht to
draw attention to the fact that he has in fact succeeded in isolating a
number of alkaloidal compounds, some of them indoles.
Mechoulam   Professor Salemink has published the isolation of a few
simple nitrogen-containing compounds which are not active in the
ranges in which they are present.
Haney   These compounds are very unstable, and quite likely they
might be altered in the processing of hashish, or destroyed altogether.
So if one were going to look for them, one had better start with
absolutely fresh plant material.
Braenden   We have also obtained some relevant information at the
United Nations Laboratory. Instead of the classical procedure using
petroleum ether for the extraction of cannabis, we applied a typical
method for the extraction of alkaloids and obtained a residue which
appeared to contain substances of an alkaloidal nature. This residue
gave positive reactions for alkaloids when treated with picric acid,
Mayer's reagent and Marme's reagent; and, with thin-layer chromatography, four spots were found after the plates were sprayed with a

reagent for alkaloids. Earlier, Professor C. A. Salemink reported the isolation of certain quarternary ammonium bases from cannabis. As such substances may be highly active pharmacologically, I consider that it is essential for this aspect of the chemistry of cannabis to be thoroughly investigated before any final conclusions are made concerning the composition of cannabis.

(g) Detection in Biological Media

A. S. Curry I wanted to take up this point of the very high pharmacological activity per unit weight of the cannabis products. I have the problem of trying to detect these materials in body fluids. I agree with Dr. Agurell's figures for urine, and think that many workers have found the same sort of order, but this is a useless figure as far as blood is concerned. Are there any developments in fluorimetric analysis? As far as I can see, this is the only hope of achieving the necessary degree of sensitivity to detect cannabis products in blood.

Paton Would it not be better to look for a metabolite rather than the active substance? Just as one approaches the problem of looking for catecholamines or 5-hydroxytryptamine in a patient.

A. S. Curry These assays are carried out fluorimetrically, in the main. The technique will have to detect picograms per mil, not nanograms per mil.

Paton If, as Professor Korte says, there is definite evidence that cannabinol is the metabolite, perhaps one ought to concentrate on detecting that in blood.

Korte I am not very good at calculations, but it is true that in the hospital it is cannabinol that can be detected most clearly in urine.

(h) Nomenclature

Crombie It might be desirable to have some agreed way of writing formulae, and some agreed numbering among those interested in cannabinols, but this may not be accepted in the wider literature of chemistry. Also, freedom to write a structure in any way the author desires must be retained; an author may be trying to emphasize a particular point.

Fairbairn Normally an author merely wants to show that four or five compounds are present in a particular situation. Is there any reason, for instance, why I should not always write about a terpene?

Crombie There is no absolute rule. It depends on the system one is using. If there were an internationally agreed system, of course one would follow this. We could seek advice about the system likely to receive most international agreement, but even then, there will still remain variations between journals.

Agurell   If the IUPAC Committee says there is a definite way for numbering, perhaps it would be reasonable to conform with that.

Crombie   I will try to find out what the IUPAC opinion would be.

Mechoulam   Two numbering systems are today usually employed, the dibenzopyran and monoterpene systems. The advantage of the dibenzopyran numbering for THC is that it is in line with the rules employed by Chemical Abstracts. Its disadvantage is that on passing from the THC series to the cannabidiol series and/or to the *iso*—THC series (or vice-versa) the numbering loses its validity. The carbon atoms in cannabidiol should be numbered in a second manner and those of an *iso*—THC in still another way.

In the monoterpene-type numbering such a constant switching-over of numbering systems will be mostly avoided. Therefore we have suggested and used this system.

As the cannabinoid field appears to be of interest to scientists of widely different specialities it is of importance to try and keep the formal difficulties in this field to a minimum. A common numbering for all cannabinoids (as in the monoterpene-type numbering) is thus to be preferred.

Joyce   The proceedings of this meeting might contain an Appendix or Glossary, giving just this kind of cross-reference. This might be of assistance, not only to the chemists, who are obviously very much at home with these problems, but also to the people whom one foresees will make use of their work. Even pharmacologists might be prevailed upon to use some kind of system of referencing when they come to do their animal or human work. At the moment, it is very difficult to compare what people at different centres of research have really done. Not only have they sometimes treated hashish as a simple substance (and we can hope, at least after the publication of the Proceedings of these two days, that they will not continue to do that), but they even refer to synthetic and presumably pure substance as though it were several different ones. I think a glossary might help to reduce that sort of confusion.

Crombie   It might be useful to decide on the most useful workaday representation.

Joyce   We cannot bind anybody but it might still be useful to make a decision of this kind.

A. S. Curry   Can we not use, in the discussions and in the papers, one nomenclature? I think pharmacologists and botanists will be greatly confused by the use of Δ^8 and $\Delta^{1\,(b)}$ for the same compound in the same meeting.

Shulgin   Todd's work of 20 years ago used yet a different nomenclature. Now, to understand his work, you have to examine his ideas about the biosynthesis and chemistry of the compounds to discover which ones he was writing about.

Paton It would be worth including a reference to Todd's nomenclature in the Appendix.

Crombie There are really two questions: Which system do the members of this gathering feel is the most generally accepted; and which is most useful to them. There are really five choices: The dibenzylpyrene representation, with two types of numbering, the diphenyl system, or the monoterpene system, which most authors have used, but there are also two types of numbering to that.

Korte The Auerbach people are responsible for nomenclature, and their suggestions will in the end prove most authoritative.

Petrzilka The Δ^8, Δ^9 nomenclature is winning support, if you take the Anglo-Saxon literature as a guide; everybody seems to prefer that for tetrahydrocannabinol.

Mechoulam What about the isotetrahydrocannabinols?

Petrzilka They are bicyclo compounds which you should number according to *Chemical Abstracts.*

Shulgin It seems that we are not going to have a unanimous vote.

Crombie The issue is, do we want a uniform nomenclature and numbering within this volume? If so, the system must be agreed upon.

Joyce Even if a uniform system were agreed upon, it would be a considerable task to carry it out. It might be best to rely upon an adequate Glossary so that those who wish can make the translations as and when they are needed.

Crombie Can we agree that ultimately the IUPAC systems will be the ones that should be employed?

Fairbairn How long would IUPAC take to decide?

Korte The members of the Commission agree upon a common nomenclature when they are sitting together, but when they return to their laboratories they publish under all kinds of different nomenclatures.

Crombie Even with IUPAC nomenclature and numbering, the pharmacologists will no doubt still refer to these compounds by their own pet systems.

When such a question goes before the correctly authorized body the amount of debate which occurs is very considerable, before a decision is reached.

Halbach Some members of the audience here may also be members of the IUPAC Committee. Perhaps they could advance some ideas of what IUPAC would say. With luck, their views may coincide.

A. S. Curry I find it difficult to believe that Lord Todd and others

did not consider this problem right at the very beginning. I wonder
why Todd's system has fallen into disuse?

Crombie   Because changes in nomenclature are continually occurring.

Fairbairn   So chemists are as bad as botanists, always changing the
species' name and transferring it to another genus, I had always
thought how nice it must be to be a chemist where everything is so
nicely set out!

Crombie   It is agreed, then, that we produce a glossary and that those
members who have presented papers shall use such systems as they
consider best.

A. S. Curry   Can we at least decide on which way up the molecule
shall be written?

Shulgin   Once you have named the compound in an acceptable way
and defined exactly what you are talking about, I think there is more
virtue in portraying the molecule in as many ways as possible instead
of in a consistent way. The entire presentation of Dr. Petrzilka would
have been impossible if he had been obliged to portray everything in
exactly the same way.

A. S. Curry   I agree, but personally I find it easier if a standard system
is used to show a reaction system.

Crombie   If you write things in different ways, different thoughts
enter your head.

Paton   If one did not have to bother about international agreement
but only the present group, which system would be preferred?

(A vote was taken on preferences for the alternative systems. Eight
preferences were expressed: three for the dibenzylpyrene system and
five for the monoterpene system—Mechoulam type).

Mechoulam   As I understand it, there are two systems for THCs: one
is the Δ^1 system and the other is the Δ^9 system. I suggest that the
terpene numbering fits all requirements.

Crombie   There is actually a difference here, because you are con-
ceiving one as a dibenzylpyrene, and the other as having a terpene
unit attached. It is when you come to the other compounds that
problems arise; this is the point I was trying to make.

A. S. Curry   I find it extremely difficult to prefer one of two logical
systems of numbering. I do not think there is a right and wrong about
this. The choice must be made by the authorised body.

Korte   Could we agree to ask IUPAC and Chemical Abstracts to tell
us which nomenclature we should use? Their advice could be added
to this publication as well, so that it is available for future use.

Joyce   I should like to do the right thing for the chemists; but I am also concerned that those who want to build upon the chemistry should be able to do it in a consistent and mutually intelligible way. This discussion has evolved guide-lines which should make something of the kind possible.

Crombie   No one would use the full nomenclature in conversation, or in ordinary writing. These are indexing matters. All that we require is a set of trivial names in order to understand each other's meanings properly.

Paton   I suppose trivial nomenclatures have a finite life, though.

Crombie   Some trivial nomenclatures in use today are very ancient, and people have found them extremely valuable, and do not talk in terms of the correct nomenclature.

In the end, I think we shall have to accept the internationally recognized chemical system, but no doubt we shall all retain our own trivial systems for use in our laboratories or amongst ourselves.

I think chemists have long been aware of all of these difficulties. What we "decide" today may eventually tie our hands if the chemistry of these compounds should take another direction.

One other point in indexing nomenclature is that capital Ds for configurations should no longer be used. This is now quite meaningless, obsolete, and archaic.

Lister   There is one argument against using the word cannabinol at all. If some of the compounds we have been talking about do in fact develop into therapeutic agents, there will be a certain opprobrium about referring to them as cannabinols of any kind. So even though they may originally have started life as cannabinols, they may end up as pyrenes or something like that.

A. S. Curry   This discussion will at least have served a very valuable purpose if it draws the attention of the soft scientists to the confusion, and to the consequent necessity to be careful about nomenclature.

(As mentioned in the Introduction, Professor Crombie was invited to summarize the present situation on nomenclature. His summary appears as an Appendix to this volume, at p. 209).

PART THREE

PHARMACOLOGICAL ASPECTS

1 Pharmacological Experiments *in vitro* on the Active Principles of Cannabis

E. W. Gill and W. D. M. Paton

Various preparations of cannabis have been given to whole animals; but there has been a notable lack of work on isolated organs or tissues, although such work is often essential for defining mechanisms of pharmacological action. This paper describes preliminary experiments, initiated in an attempt to find some suitable pharmacological response *in vitro,* on which further analysis of action might be based. It was also hoped that light might be thrown on the question of whether the action of cannabis is attributable to one, or more than one, active principle.

THE PREPARATIONS OF CANNABIS USED

The earliest experiments were made with tincture of cannabis. But, although effects could be obtained which were not attributable to ethanol, the action of the latter was detectable on the preparations used in concentrations of 1 mg/ml upwards, and obviously made analytic work impossible. The following purification method was therefore adopted.

Tincture of Cannabis B.P.C. was freed from ethanol by evaporation at 30°C *in vacuo.* The dark green viscous residue was divided into "petrol-soluble" and "petrol-insoluble" fractions by shaking vigorously with petroleum spirit (b.p. 60-80°C) for 20 min in a mechanical shaker, decanting the petrol solution from the viscous residue and removing the solvent *in vacuo.* Approximately 45% of the crude cannabis extract was soluble in petrol. Saline extracts of these two fractions (termed "petrol-insoluble" and "petrol-soluble" respectively)

were obtained by shaking with saline in a high-speed mechanical
shaker for 20 min and were then filtered.

The petrol-soluble fraction was further purified by column
chromatography and counter-current distribution, essentially as
described by Korte and Sieper (1960). Cannabinoids were obtained
by eluting an alumina column successively with petroleum spirit,
petroleum and 20% diethyl ether, and finally pure ether. The
fractions eluted by these solvents were kept separate; thin layer
chromatography showed that they were all overlapping mixtures.
Fraction III, the ether eluate, contained the more polar components
and was not purified further. Fraction II (petroleum spirit + 20%
ether) was further purified by counter-current distribution using the
system petroleum spirit (60-80); methanol; water: 10; 9; 1. After
150 transfers the distribution of cannabinoids was determined by
measuring absorbance at 280 mμ and at least 4 components could
be detected. Tubes containing the third component (partition constant $K = 0.72$) were pooled, and the product purified by a further
150 transfers. A single major peak (referred to as fraction IIc) was
obtained, which ran as a single component on thin layer chromatography and which had an infra-red spectrum identical with that of
Δ^1-tetrahydrocannabinol published by Mechoulam and Gaoni (1967).

For use, a saline extract of each fraction was made up to the volume of tincture from which it derived, and doses are therefore in
terms of 'tincture equivalent'. In every case, the saline extraction left
a considerable residue. The tincture consists of 5% extract of cannabis
resin in alcohol, but the constitution of the resin used by the suppliers
is not known quantitatively. In general, the amounts of the active
substances present are, therefore, unknown; but in the case of fraction
IIc, a saline extract was estimated spectrophotometrically to contain
approximately (and not more than) 7 μg/ml Δ^1-tetrahydrocannabinol.

PHARMACOLOGICAL METHODS

The general pharmacology of cannabis suggests, in its various aspects,
analogies with the properties of cocaine (euphoria and certain sympa-
thomimetic effects), amphetamine (in the same way, together with
the interaction between the drugs), morphine (euphoria and, reputedly,
analgesia), LSD (sensory disturbances), atropine or hyoscine (tachy-
cardia), and possibly alcohol; the chemical structure of Δ^1-tetrahydro-

cannabinol, with its phenolic hydroxyl group, recalls certain features of morphine and catecholamine structure. The preparations were chosen, therefore, so that each of the drugs named would have been detectable; in addition, there were the general considerations that it could be useful to study both an adrenergic and a cholinergic neuro-effector, and that smooth muscle preparations are, generally speaking, sensitive in one way or another to most drugs of synaptic interest. The two preparations chosen, therefore, were:

(a) guinea-pig vas deferens, excited by field stimulation (10-50 V/cm voltage gradient) with single shocks of 1 msec duration every 30 or 60 sec. The vas deferens is customarily stimulated with trains of shocks; but since (for instance) the depressant action of morphine on acetylcholine liberated by Auerbach's plexus virtually disappears at frequencies above 1-3/sec, it was decided that single shocks should be used, although a response was only obtained if strong field stimulation was employed. The responses obtained are therefore *not* equivalent to those normally described.

(b) guinea-pig ileum, excited by field stimulation (1-5 V/cm gradient) with single shocks of 1 msec duration every 10-30 sec.

Each preparation was mounted in a 7 ml bath, maintained at 37°C, filled with Krebs-Henseleit solution, bubbled with 5% CO_2/95% O_2. Washout was by overflow. Stimuli were delivered through platinum electrodes suitably placed above and below the preparation. The longitudinal contractions of the vas or ileum (up to 5 g tension) were recorded isometrically with an RCA transducer and servo-pen recorder. Stimulation was intermitted as required when the response to direct acting drugs was tested.

RESULTS

(a) *The petrol-insoluble fraction.* On the stimulated guinea-pig ileum this fraction depressed both the twitch response to electrical stimulation, and the direct response to acetylcholine (Fig. 1a). The antagonism to acetylcholine appeared to be competitive, as shown by a parallel shift of the log-dose-response curve (Fig. 1b). A dose-ratio of approximately 7-fold was produced by 0.3 ml of the petrol-insoluble fraction. The effect was reversible, half recovery occurring in about 5 min. This intensity of antagonism is, by comparison with known specific antagonists such as atropine, sufficient to account

for the reduction of the twitch. There appears, therefore, to be
an atropine-like substance in the petrol-insoluble fraction.

(b) *Fraction III.* In contrast, fraction III also depressed the
response of the ileum to stimulation and to acetylcholine, but not

(*a*)

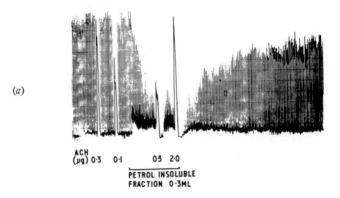

Fig. 1. (a) Response of guinea-pig ileum to field stimulation at
1/10 sec, and during intermission, to acetylcholine (ACH) 0.1, 0.3
and 2.0 μg. Saline extract of petrol-insoluble fraction, 0.3 ml.,
depresses both responses.

(b) Graph of responses to acetylcholine against log dose of
petrol-insoluble fraction, from 1(a).

(*b*)

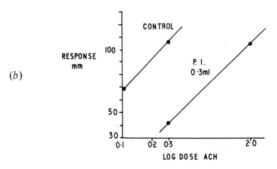

in a competitive manner. In Fig. 2, with 0.5 ml the twitch declined
by more than 50%; the response to 0.05 μg acetylcholine was unaf-
fected, although responses to 0.1 μg and 0.2 μg were substantially
reduced. The effect on the twitch was reversible, but rather slowly.

KREBS : 37°C : 5%CO$_2$/95%O$_2$: 7 ML BATH.

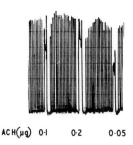

ACH(µg) 0·1   0·2   0·05

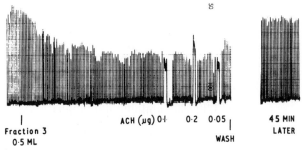

	ACH (µg) 0·1 0·2 0·05		45 MIN
Fraction 3		WASH	LATER
0·5 ML			

Fig. 2. As Fig. 1(a), showing effect of Fraction III.

KREBS : 5%CO$_2$/95%O$_2$: 37°C
7 ML BATH

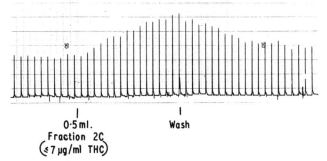

0·5 ml.   Wash
Fraction 2C
(⩽7 µg/ml THC)

Fig. 3. Response of guinea-pig vas deferens to field stimulation
of 1/min. Potentiation by Fraction IIc (approximately 7 µg/ml
Δ^1-THC), 0.5 ml, followed by recovery on washing out.

The effect has not been analysed, but resembles the non-specific effect of alcohols.

(c) *Fraction IIc.* The most interesting results were obtained with this fraction, which was indistinguishable from pure Δ^1-tetrahydro-

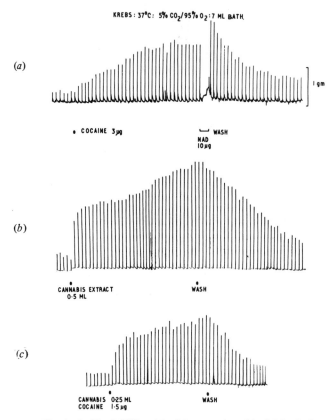

KREBS : 37°C: 5% CO_2/95% O_2 : 7 ML BATH

(a)

I gm

• COCAINE 3 µg   WASH
NAD
10 µg

(b)

CANNABIS EXTRACT   WASH
0·5 ML

(c)

CANNABIS 0·25 ML   WASH
COCAINE 1·5 µg

Fig. 4. As Fig. 3. Effect (a) of 3 µg cocaine, (b) of 0.5 ml of petrol-soluble fraction and (c) of 0.25 ml petrol-soluble fraction combined with 1.5 µg cocaine, showing additive effect of the two drugs.

cannabinol. On the vas deferens, a potentiation of the twitch is produced by doses from 0.1 ml upwards. The effect is of gradual onset, although usually detectable in 1-2 min (Fig. 3). On washing out, it passes off with roughly the same time course. For any given dose, it seems possible that the effect is limited by uptake of the drug; since

if the bath is washed out, and the same dose replaced, a further incre-
ment in the response occurs. Fig. 4a shows that a similar potentiation
of the twitch can be produced with cocaine. In this particular experiment, Fraction IIc was not yet available, and a simple saline extract

KREBS : 37°C : 5%CO$_2$/95% O$_2$: 7 ML BATH

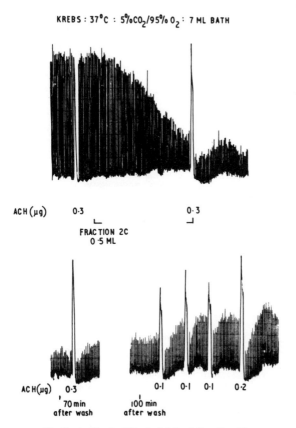

Fig. 5. As Fig. 1. Effect of 0.5 ml Fraction IIc.

of the whole petrol-soluble fraction was used (free of ethanol); this
extract exerted the same effect, although with a more prompt initial
phase (Fig. 4b). Fig. 4c shows a test for mutual synergism or potentiation, in which half-doses of each drug are combined; the resultant
response is intermediate between the two control responses, and provides evidence for a simple summation of effect between cocaine and

the extract. No consistent potentiation of noradrenaline was obtained; but it must be remembered that the vas is notoriously insensitive to externally applied catecholamine.

On the ileum, fraction IIc produced a gradual but profound depression of the twitch response to electrical stimulation, without affecting the response to added acetylcholine (Fig. 5). In this respect

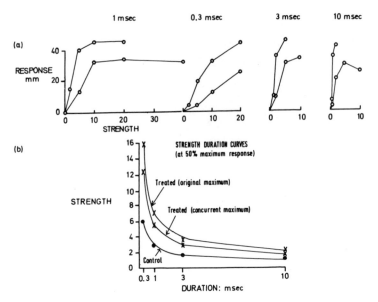

Fig. 6. (a) Graphs of response of guinea-pig ileum to field stimulation at various strengths, for shock duration of 0.3, 1, 3 and 10 msec, before (upper curves in each panel) and after (lower curves) treatment with 0.5 ml Fraction IIc.
(b) Strength-duration curves derived from (a).

it resembles morphine and the opiates (Paton, 1957); but it is dissimilar in the extraordinary persistence of the effect, recovery being far from complete 120 min after washing out the drug. Treatment with acetylcholine seemed slightly to accelerate recovery, but choline did not.

Further experiments provided evidence that this effect was in part due to a reduction in excitability of the nerve fibres of the ileum. Fig. 6a shows strength-response curves for various stimulus durations before and after treatment with fraction IIc. At all durations, the curve is shifted to the right, and the maximum response depressed. Fig. 6b shows the strength-duration curves derived. Since the maximum response was depressed, the curves have been drawn for the chosen level (50% maximum taken either for the control maximum, or for the maximum under the influence of the extract).

CONCLUSIONS

These preliminary experiments show (1) that pharmacological actions of cannabis are demonstrable on *in vitro* preparations;

(2) that at least three active principles are present, provisionally compared with atropine, with an alcohol, and with morphine or cocaine. These comparisons are purely operational, and may well be misleading ultimately as regards the mechanism of action.

(3) The most interesting action is that of Δ^1-tetrahydrocannabinol. This is exerted at a concentration of the order of 10^{-6} g/ml; it may well represent the *in vitro* counterpart of the physiologically active principle.

References

Korte, F. and Sieper, H., *Annalen* 630:71 (1960).
Mechoulam, R. and Gaone, T., *Fortschr. Chem. Org. Naturstoffe* 25:175 (1967).
Paton, W. D. M., *Brit. J. Pharmacol.* 12:119 (1957).

2 Chemical and Pharmacological Studies of Cannabis

Stig Agurell

with the participation of Inger Nilsson, J. Lars, G. Nilsson, Agneta Ohlsson, Kerstin Olofsson, Finn Sandberg and Marianne Wahlqvist of the Faculty of Pharmacy and Jan-Erik Lindgren of the Department of Toxicology, Karolinska Institute Stockholm.

ANALYSIS OF BIOLOGICAL SAMPLES FOR CANNABIS CONSTITUENTS

Pharmacological studies suggest that the tetrahydrocannabinols are the centrally active constituents. In particular it appears that Δ^1-tetrahydrocannabinol may be the major active compound (Weil, Zinberg and Nelsen, 1968; Isbell, Gorodetzky, Jasinski, Claussen, Spulak and Korte, 1967; Scheckel, Boff, Dahlen and Smart, 1968). However, recent data suggest (Weil *et al.*, 1968; Claussen and Korte, 1968) that the dose of Δ^1-tetrahydrocannabinol necessary to give psychological effects in man, when smoked, may be as low as 2-3 μg/kg. The possibility of working out chemical tests for the detection of Cannabis use would thus have to rely on extremely sensitive and selective means of identification.

The isolation, separation, and identification of Cannabis constituents by various methods was reviewed by Grlic in 1964. Two suitable methods for identification are thin-layer chromatography (Agurell *et al.*, 1969a; Korte and Sieper, 1964; Parker, Wright, Halpern and Hine, 1968) and, in particular, gas chromatography (Agurell *et al.*, 1969b; Parker *et al.*, 1968; among others). It is generally accepted that gas chromatographic procedures for the analysis of drugs, when applicable, surpass other methods particularly in sensitivity. A comparison between the detection limits would suggest about 1 μg for thin-layer chromatography (Parker *et al.*, 1968) and

175

about 1 ng for gas chromatography (FID). It is quite possible that amounts of cannabinols even below the ng level may be estimated and identified by gas chromatography of e.g. heptafluorobutyrate derivatives using electron capture detection (Exley, 1968).

In the model experiments (Agurell *et al.,* 1969*a, b*) designed to test methods for the identification of Cannabis users, rats (200 g) were given non-labelled cannabinols (50 mg/kg; 71% tetrahydrocannabinol) i.p. Urine was collected for 24 hr periods, saturated with NaCl and extracted three times with an equal volume of light petroleum and

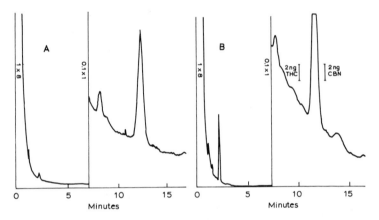

Fig. 1. Gas chromatogram of purified light petroleum extract of urine from control rat (A); and rat injected with cannabinols (50 mg/kg) i.p. (B). Retention time and approx. peak height for 2 ng Δ^1-tetrahydrocannabinol (THC) and cannabinol (CBN) indicated.

dried (Na$_2$SO$_4$). The light petroleum extract was subjected to a further purification by thin-layer chromatography on Silica Gel H with 12% ether in hexane as solvent. All three cannabinols have close R$_f$ values in this system. The area corresponding to the R$_f$ values of the cannabinols was removed from the plate and eluted with ether. The eluate was analyzed by gas chromatography (Fig. 1), without detecting any cannabinols.

Estimating a lower detection limit of 2 ng tetrahydrocannabinol in the gas chromatographic identification step, it may be calculated that at most 0.005% of the introduced cannabinols were excreted unchanged in urine during the first 24 hours.

Experiments with cannabidiol (28-250 ng) added to urine showed recovery from the extraction—thin-layer chromatographic procedure to be about 70%.

Parker *et al.,* (1968) suggested a similar scheme for the determination of tetrahydrocannabinol added to urine. They utilized an initial chloroform extraction followed, without further purification, by gas chromatographic analysis. A lower detection limit of 10 ng tetrahydrocannabinol per ml urine is indicated, similar to our results described above.

Mass fragmentography   Recently, instruments combining gas chromatography with mass spectrometry have been made commercially available. In these instruments a separation system of high selectivity

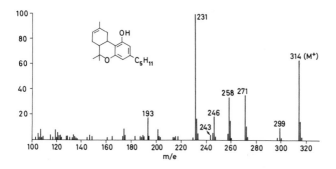

Fig. 2. Mass spectrum of $\Delta^{1(6)}$-tetrahydrocannabinol.

(GLC column) and a simple means of identification (retention time) are combined with an excellent means of structural identification (mass spectrum). Potentially it would be very valuable in identifying tetrahydrocannabinol, or metabolites thereof, in the urine or blood plasma of Cannabis users. However, to obtain a mass spectrum, about 1 μg of compound is needed. This is probably a higher amount than one can expect in biological samples.

By the use of a slightly different technique involving an Accelerating Voltage Alternator (AVA) unit with the LKB 9,000 gas chromatograph-mass spectrometer, the sensitivity can be increased about 1,000 times although at the cost of less information. This technique was introduced by Sweeley, Elliott, Fries and Ryhage (1966) and has been developed for the identification of minute amounts of drugs by

Hammar, Holmstedt, Lindgren and Tham (1969). These authors have also discussed in detail the technical aspects.

In principle, the mass spectrometer is used continuously to monitor three mass numbers of compounds eluted from the gas chromatograph. The recording of the three mass numbers in the effluate resembles an ordinary gas chromatogram. In Fig. 2 is shown the mass spectrum of $\Delta^{1(6)}$-tetrahydrocannabinol. Fragments m/e 231 (base peak), 243 and 246 from 80 and 8 ng respectively of Δ^1-tetrahydrocannabinol in the eluate of the gas chromatograph are shown in Figure 3. This technique, called "mass fragmentography" by Hammar

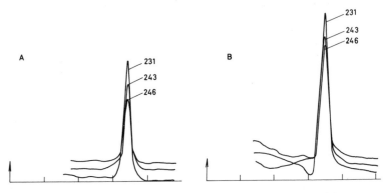

Fig. 3. Mass fragmentogram of (A) 80 ng, (B) 8 ng (max. sensitivity) Δ^1-tetrahydrocannabinol. Focusing upon fragments m/e 231, 243 (signal multiplied 2 times) and 246 (signal multiplied 4 times). Arrow shows time of injection; time scale in minutes. Column temperature 240°; 5% SE-30 on Gas Chrom P.

et al. (1969) thus provides retention time and a partial mass spectrum. By repeated focusing on several different fragments a more complete mass spectrum may be obtained. This technique is now being used by us to investigate urine and blood plasma from Cannabis users.

LABELLED CANNABINOLS

Metabolic studies on Cannabis constituents in man and experimental animals have long been hampered by the lack of labelled compounds necessary to investigate the metabolic fate of these most potent entities. Miras (1965) produced small amounts of tetrahydrocanna-

binol-C^{14} by growing Cannabis plants in $C^{14}O_2$. Recently Burstein
and Mechoulam (1968) elegantly prepared specifically tritium labelled
$\Delta^{1(6)}$-tetrahydrocannabinol by isomerization of Δ^1-tetrahydrocanna-
binol in the presence of p-toluenesulphonic acid.

Since we had extensive experience of labelling phenols in tritiated
water by acid catalysis, we investigated this method to obtain tritium

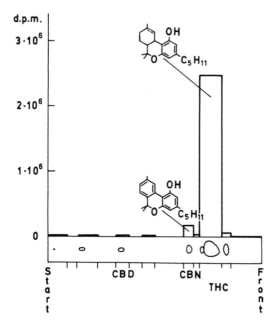

Fig. 4. Distribution of radioactivity, determined by liquid scintillation counting, on thin-layer chromatogram of Δ^1-tetrahydro-
cannabinol-H^3 (THC) before purification by TLC. Three per cent
of the radioactivity present in cannabinol (CBN; cannabidiol
(CBD).

labelled tetrahydrocannabinol, as follows: 50 mg Δ^1-tetrahydrocan-
nabinol; 0.5 ml phosphoric acid; 2.5 ml tetrahydrofuran and 0.25 ml
tritiated water were heated under nitrogen to 80° for 30 min. After
removal of exchangeable hydrogens and purification by thin-layer
chromatography (Parker *et al.,* 1968), Δ^1-tetrahydrocannabinol with
specific activities of up to 12 mC/mM was obtained (Agurell *et al.,*
1969*a, b*). The product was shown by thin-layer chromatography and

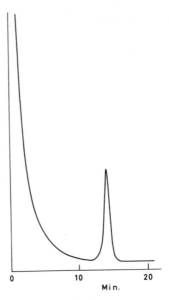

Fig. 5. Gas chromatogram of Δ^1-tetrahydrocannabinol-H^3 purified by TLC SE-30 column. Temp. 225°. By comparison with reference compounds shown to be free from the $\Delta^{1(6)}$-isomer.

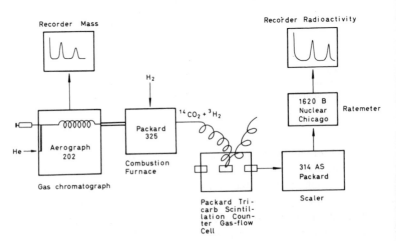

Fig. 6. Flow diagram of instruments for radiochromatography.

gas chromatography (Petrzilka and Sikemeier, 1967) on an SE-30 column to consist of pure or almost pure Δ^1-tetrahydrocannabinol (Fig. 4 and 5). The label was shown to be stable in biological systems, but gas chromatography (250°C) of methanolic solution of Δ^1-tetra-

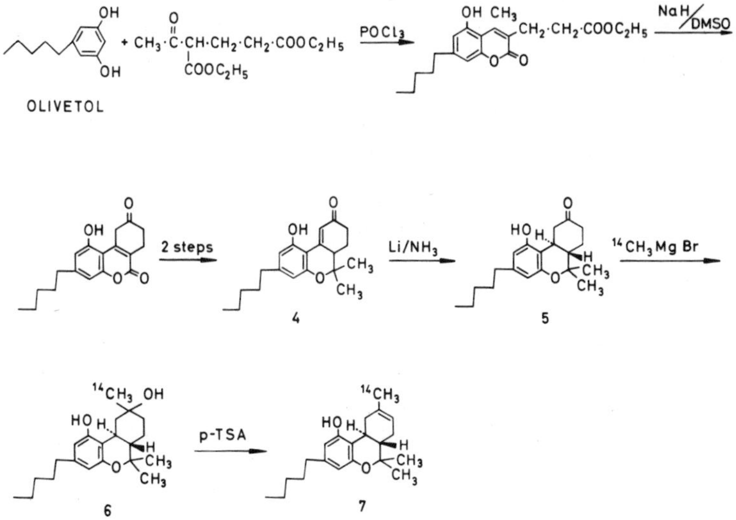

Fig. 7. Synthesis of $\Delta^{1(6)}$-tetrahydrocannabinol-C^{14}. This compound may be converted to the Δ^1-isomer. (T. Petrzilka and C. Sikemeier, Helv. Chim. Acta, 50:2111, 1967). After reduction of the unsaturated ketone (4) with Li/NH$_3$(20), the cis- and trans-ketones were separated and 100 mg of the trans-ketone (5) was acetylated as described (20). It was then treated with methyl-magnesium bromide (from 350 mg CH$_3$Br; 1 mC^{14}C) in ether and after the usual work up procedure, the tertiary alcohol (6) was isolated as an oil. This oil was dissolved in 100 ml of benzene, 10 mg of p-toluene sulphonic acid was added and the solution was refluxed for 4 hrs. From this reaction 43 mg of $\Delta^{1(6)}$-tetra-hydrocannabinol holding an activity of 470 μC/mM was isolated as an oil by preparative TLC. The identity of the compound was established by chromatographic and spectral comparison with authentic material.

hydrocannabinol-H^3 followed by simultaneous analysis of the mass (T.C.) and radioactivity (Packard Combustion Furnace; gas flow cell; Packard Scintillation Counter) of the eluate showed that the label exchanged completely in the chromatograph, appearing with the solvent front and thereby definitely complicating the structural elucidation of metabolites. It is our hope that this analyzer unit for radiochromatography will facilitate metabolic studies with C^{14}-labelled cannabinols (Fig. 6).

For this reason and also for technical purposes related to the counting of radioactive samples, we considered it preferable to prepare C^{14}-labelled tetrahydrocannabinol. The subsequent chemical work has been carried out by Dr. J. L. G. Nilsson, and essentially is in accordance with the total synthesis of dl-Δ^1-tetrahydrocannabinol described by Fahrenholtz, Lurie and Kierstad (1967). The synthetic sequence is shown in Fig. 7 and the label is introduced by the use of $C^{14}H_3Br$ in the final Grignard reaction.

Two other labelling procedures are under investigation, both relying on the condensation of labelled olivetol with p-menthadienol as described by Petrzilka and Sikemeier (1967). In one case 3,5-dimethoxybenzaldehyde is reacted in a Grignard reaction with butyl iodide to yield dimethyl olivetol containing, in addition, a benzylic hydroxyl group in the side chain. Elimination of water followed by reduction of the exocyclic double bond with tritium gas and demethylation would be expected to yield inexpensive olivetol of high specific activity, labelled in the side chain. The other procedure involves the synthesis of olivetol from ethyl acetoacetate-3-C^{14} (Korte and Sieper, 1960).

ELIMINATION AND DISTRIBUTION OF TETRAHYDROCANNABINOL-H^3 IN THE RABBIT

We have previously shown that intravenously injected tetrahydrocannabinol-H^3 is eliminated very slowly by the rat (Agurell *et al.*, 1969). About half of the administered drug still remained in the body after one week and about 8% of the drug was excreted in the faeces. We have now carried out similar and other studies in the rabbit.

The elimination of Δ^1-tetrahydrocannabinol-H^3 in the rabbit (Fig. 8) differs greatly from that in the rat. In the rabbit, the major elimination is by the kidneys, about 30% of the adminstered drug being excreted during the first 24 hrs. This is in contrast to only a few per cent in the rat. A detailed investigation of the radioactivity in the urine by extraction with light petroleum and ether as in the previous study with rats, indicated that at most 0.01% of the introduced tetrahydrocannabinol-H^3 was excreted as such in the urine

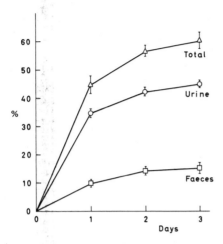

Fig. 8. Elimination of radioactivity in the rabbit from Δ^1-tetra-hydrocannabinol-H³. Four rabbits given 72×10^6-157×10^6 d.p.m./kg or 0.4-1.1 mg/kg. Mean values with standard deviations.

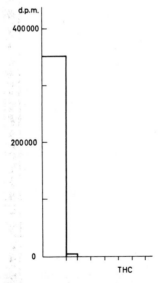

Fig. 9. Distribution of radioactivity in ether extract of urine from rabbit given Δ^1-tetrahydrocannabinol-H³. TLC on dimethyl-formamide treated Silica gel G; 20% ether in light petroleum. R_F value of tetrahydrocannabinol indicated.

during the first 24 hrs. A considerable amount of the activity remaining in the urine (Fig. 9) could be extracted with ether (4-7%).

In Fig. 10 the elimination of Δ^1-tetrahydrocannabinol-H^3 is compared in rat, rabbit and man. In the latter case a small amount (56 μg 2.1 μC) was administered orally, and direct comparison is therefore difficult. However, it is evident that a considerable part of the drug is eliminated by the kidneys in man.

We also investigated the half life of Δ^1-tetrahydrocannabinol-H^3 in rabbit blood after i.v. injection. Blood samples were taken at

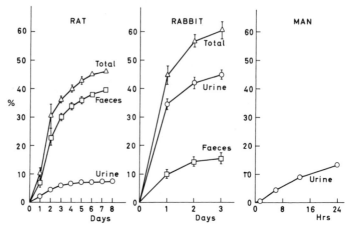

Fig. 10. Excretion of radioactivity from Δ^1-tetrahydrocannabinol-H^3 in rat (four rats: 1.3 mg/kg; 285 x 10^6 d.p.m. kg i.v. injection), rabbit (four rabbits; 0.4-1.1 mg/kg; 72-157 x 10^6 d.p.m./kg; i.v. injection) and man (mean of two experiments; 56 μg; 4.6 x 10^6 d.p.m.; orally). Mean values and standard deviations shown. Please note different time scales.

intervals from the ear and the amount of radioactivity remaining determined. The results in Fig. 11 indicate a half life of radioactivity in the blood of about 14 min. The half life value from five experiments ranged between 7-16 min.

It should be noted that after 30 minutes only a few per cent (3-4% in three different experiments) of the radioactivity is present as tetrahydrocannabinol. Extraction of blood samples from different time intervals with light petroleum and ether, as described for urine, showed a rapid formation of an ether soluble metabolite as well as

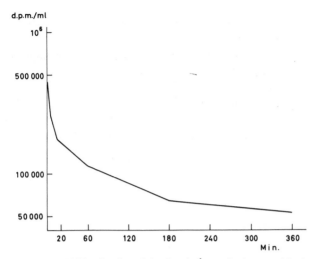

Fig. 11. Half-life of radioactivity from Δ^1-tetrahydrocannabinol-H^3 in blood of rabbit after i.v. injection; 0.3 mg/kg; 92 x 10^6 d.p.m./kg.

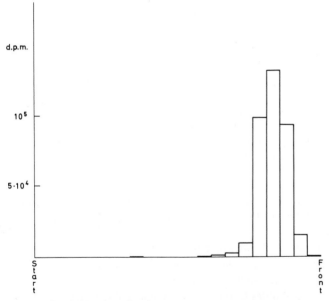

Fig. 12. Distribution of radioactivity on paper chromatogram. Ether soluble metabolite(s) of Δ^1-tetrahydrocannabinol-H^3 from rabbit urine; *n*-butanol-acetic acid-water (4:1:5).

more water soluble products. The formation of an active metabolite therefore cannot be excluded.

So far we have found no particularly suitable separation system for the separation and isolation of the ether soluble metabolite. However, we have not been able to distinguish by paper chromatography in n-butanol-acetic acid-water (4:1:5), the ether soluble metabolite(s) from the urine of rat or rabbit from the metabolite in the blood of rabbit or from the product obtained by incubating Δ^1-tetrahydrocannabinol-H^3 with the "10,000 g supernatant" from rat liver (Fig. 12).

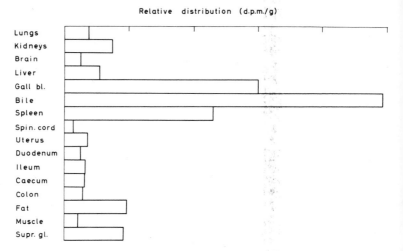

Fig. 13. Relative distribution of radioactivity in the rabbit three days after i.v. injection of Δ^1-tetrahydrocannabinol-H^3 (mean of four animals). Blood level slightly less than level in muscle.

The relative distribution (d.p.m./g tissue) of radioactivity in the rabbit (mean of four rabbits) three days after injection of Δ^1-tetrahydrocannabinol-H^3 is shown in Fig. 13. In general, it may be noted that brain and spinal cord contain little activity and that muscular tissues contain less activity than fat, where the lipophilic drug would be expected to accumulate to a certain extent. The elimination of radioactive metabolites through liver and bile is also evident (note that the contents of the small intestines were removed before activity determination). A striking observation is the relatively high activity present

in the spleen. Preliminary studies on the distribution of radioactivity
in the rabbit 2 hrs after injection with Δ^1-tetrahydrocannabinol-H^3
show, in general, a similar distribution as after three days, with the
following exceptions: lungs and, in particular, kidneys contain a high
amount of radioactivity while spleen and body fat contain only
little activity.

IN VITRO OXIDATION OF Δ^1-TETRAHYDROCANNABINOL-H^3

We used, in general, the *in vitro* system described by Tagg, Yasuda,
Tanabe and Mitoma (1967). Adult male rats, pretreated with sodium
phenobarbitone, were sacrificed and the livers removed. Homogenates
of liver were prepared in 2 volumes of 1.15% KCl and centrifuged
for 10 min. at 10,000 g.

TABLE 1. *Metabolism of Δ^1-tetrahydrocannabinol-H^3 (THC-H^3)*
by subcellular fraction of rat liver

Expt. No.	Unchanged THC-H^3 %	"Ether soluble metabolite" %
1A	5	28
1B	11	34
1C control*	21	1
2A	5	13
2B control*	50	1

* "10,000 g supernatant" boiled for 1 min.

The "10,000 g supernatant", 1.0 ml. was incubated for 2 hrs with
0.5 μM Δ^1-tetrahydrocannabinol-H^3, 15 μM nicotinamide, 0.25 μM
NADP, 40 μM glucose-6-phosphate, 20 μM $MgCl_2$ in 1.0 ml M/15
phosphate buffer (pH 7.0) as described by Tagg *et al.* (1967).

The incubation mixture was extracted three times with light
petroleum, followed by three extractions with ether. The amount of
radioactivity in both extracts was determined. Each extract was then
chromatographed on Silica gel G (Agurell *et al.*, 1969a, b) and the distribution of radioactivity was established. This was necessary since the
ether extract also contained some unchanged tetrahydrocannabinol.

In seven experiments, the *in vitro* system was found to convert
13-38% of added tritium-labelled tetrahydrocannabinol to an ether
soluble metabolite. This metabolite may be the same as that isolated

from rat and rabbit urine as well as from rabbit blood after administration of tetrahydrocannabinol-H^3 (Fig. 12 and Table 1).

Subcellular fractions of rat liver can thus readily metabolize
Δ^1-tetrahydrocannabinol to possibly the same metabolite(s) as are
occurring in the urine.

BINDING OF Δ^1-TETRAHYDROCANNABINOL TO PLASMA PROTEINS

Interactions between drugs and proteins are known to greatly influence
the behaviour of drugs in the body. In particular, the binding of drugs
by plasma proteins has been extensively investigated as discussed in
a recent comprehensive review (Meyer and Guttman, 1968). Methods
of detecting, determination and study of protein binding have also
been reviewed by Meyer and Guttman (1968). Protein binding influences drug concentration in tissue fluids, drug excretion, therapeutic
activity and toxicity of drugs and penetration through biological
membranes.

Our experiments on the *in vitro* oxidation of Δ^1-tetrahydrocan-
nabinol with "10,000 g supernatant" indicated that the drug might
be bound to plasma proteins. We have now made a preliminary investigation of its protein binding using ultrafiltration and disc electrophoresis.

Ultra filtration   The technique used was that described by Borga,
Azarnoff, Forshell and Sjoqvist (1969). Human blood was collected
in heparinized tubes and centrifuged to obtain the plasma.

Five ml of blood plasma or, in control experiments, M/15 phosphate buffer of pH 7.4 was incubated for 1 hr at 37° with 0.02-0.05
μM of Δ^1-tetrahydrocannabinol-H^3 dissolved in 100 μl propylene
glycol.

Each incubation mixture was enclosed in dialysis tubing and the
U-shaped bag was secured by a stopper with the bottom of the bag
3 cm above the bottom of a centrifuge tube. The tube was centrifuged for 10 min at 800 g. The dialysis bag was wiped free from
moisture and again centrifuged for 45 min at 800 g to yield a few
hundred μl of ultrafiltrate. The amount of radioactivity (d.p.m./μl)
in the ultrafiltrate compared to the d.p.m./μl in the incubation
mixture, indicates the amount of unbound drug: if a drug is not
bound to proteins the d.p.m./μl in the incubation mixture and in the

ultrafiltrate will be the same. A control sample is included to measure
the binding of the drug to the dialysis tubing.

In eight experiments the mean percentages of radioactivity in the
ultrafiltrate as compared to the incubation mixture (100%) were as
follows:

> buffer   14% (range 8-17%)
> plasma   1% (range 1-3%)

The quantitative significance of these figures is questionable since
tetrahydrocannabinol appears not to be completely dissolved in the
buffer. However, the results clearly indicate that Δ^1-tetrahydrocan-
nabinol is to a large extent bound to plasma proteins.

Disc electrophoresis   Polyacrylamide-gel electrophoresis was carried
out as described for human serum proteins by Davis (1964) with the

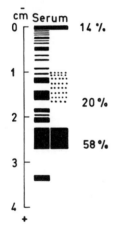

Fig. 14. Polyacrylamide gel electrophoresis of human plasma
incubated with Δ^1-tetrahydrocannabinol-H^3. Left: protein distribution. Right: distribution of radioactivity.

modifications given by Sjoholm and Yman (1966). Human plasma
(2 ml) was incubated with 0.05 μM of Δ^1-tetrahydrocannabinol-H^3
dissolved in a minimal amount of propylene glycol. Of the incubation
mixture, 10-20 μl samples were separated by disc electrophoresis.
After electrophoresis, the gels were cut longitudinally. Only half
was stained for proteins (Davis, 1964). The other half was cut into
2 mm slices and the radioactivity in each segment was determined
by liquid scintillation counting.

Analysis of the plasma proteins showed that the major part i.e. 55-58% (two experiments) of Δ^1-tetrahydrocannabinol-H^3 was present in the albumin area while 14-19% remained at the origin (Fig. 14). Disc electrophoresis of Δ^1-tetrahydrocannabinol itself showed that this compound remained mainly at the origin with the rest spread over the first 10 mm of the gel.

In this connection, it should be added that electrophoresis of rabbit plasma three hours after i.v. injection of Δ^1-tetrahydrocannabinol-H^3 still showed the major part of the activity to be associated with the albumin fraction. At this time very little of the radioactivity is present as the unchanged compound. This indicates that a major metabolite (or several minor ones) are also bound to plasma proteins.

Thus, these experiments show that tetrahydrocannabinol is mainly bound to the plasma proteins.

Acknowledgement   For valuable discussions weare indebted to Drs. C. G. Hammar, R. Hessling and L. Yman. Reference materials were kindly provided by Drs. R. Mechoulam, G. Krook and T. Petrzilka. This research was supported by the Swedish Medical Research Council (K69-13X-2724-01A).

References

Agurell, S., Holmstedt, B., Lindgren, J. E. and Schultes, R. E., *Acta Chem. Scand.* 23:903 (1969*a*).

Agurell, S., Nilsson, I., Ohlsson, A. and Sandberg, F., *Biochem. Pharmacol.* 18:1195 (1969*b*).

Borga, G., Azarnoff, D. L., Forshell, G. P. and Sjoqvist, F., *Biochem. Pharmacol.* 18:2135 (1969).

Burstein, S. and Mechoulam, R., *J. Amer. Chem. Soc.* 90:2420 (1968).

Claussen, U. and Korte, F., *Ann.* 713:162 (1968).

Claussen, U. and Korte, F., *Ann.* 713:166 (1968).

Davis, B. J., *Ann. N.Y. Acad. Sci.* 121:404 (1964).

Exley, D., *Biochem. J.* 107:285 (1968).

Fahrenholtz, K. E., Lurie, M. and Kierstad. R. W., *J. Amer. Chem. Soc.* 89:5934 (1967).

Grlic, L., *Bull. Narcotics.* 16, No. 4, 29 (1964).

Hammar, C. G., Holmstedt, B., Lindgren, J. E. and Tham R., *Adv. in Pharmacol.* in press (1969).

Isbell, H., Gorodetzky, C. W., Jasinski, D., Claussen, U., Spulak, F. and Korte, F., *Psychopharmacologia* 11:184 (1967).

Korte, F. and Sieper, H., *Ann.* 630:71 (1960).

Korte, F. and Sieper, H., *J. Chromatog.* 13:90 (1964).

Mechoulam, R. and Gaoni, Y., *Tetrahedron* 21:1223 (1965).

Meyer, M. C. and Guttman, D. E., *J. Pharm. Sci.* 57:895 (1968).

Miras, C. J., *Hashish: Its Chemistry and Pharmacology* (eds.
  G. E. W. Wolstenholme and J. Knight) Churchill, London 1965.

Parker, K. D., Wright, J. A., Halpern, A. F. and Hine, C. H., *Bull.
  Narcotics* 20, No. 4, 9 (1968).

Petrzilka, T. and Sikemeier, C., *Helv. Chim. Acta* 50:1416 (1967).

Scheckel, C. L., Boff, E., Dahlen, P. and Smart, T., *Science* 160:1467
  (1968).

Schultz, O. E. and Hoffner, G., *Arch. Pharm.* 293:1 (1960).

Sjoholm, I. and Yman, L., *Acta Pharm. Suecia* 3:377 (1966).

Sweeley, C. C., Elliott, W. H., Fries, I. and Ryhage, R., *Anal. Chem.*
  38:1549 (1966).

Tagg, J., Yasuda, D. M., Tanable, M. and Mitoma, C., *Biochem.
  Pharmacol.* 16:143 (1967).

Valle, J. R., Lapa, A. J. and Barros, G. G., *J. Pharm. Pharmacol.*
  20:798 (1968).

Weil, A. T., Zinberg, N. E. and Nelsen, J. M., *Science* 162:1234
  (1968).

3 The Marihuana Programme of the Centre for Studies of Narcotic and Drug Abuse, N.I.M.H.

John A. Scigliano and Coy W. Waller

The National Institute of Mental Health has been charged with the responsibility of determining the long-term effects of marihuana in man by the Congress and the President of the United States. The agency designated for the development and administration of the program was the Department of Health, Education and Welfare and specifically the Centre for Studies of Narcotic and Drug Abuse which is in the National Institute of Mental Health.

Because only small quantities of Δ^9-tetrahydrocannabinol (Δ^9-THC) had been produced by the early efforts of the organic chemists, when the National Institute of Mental Health initiated its programme in 1968 it was deemed necessary to plan for large quantities. This "crash" programme had as its initial phase the production of large quantities of plant material, of synthetic Δ^9-THC and of a plant extract. The lack in earlier biological studies of fully characterized materials did not permit the unequivocal statement that Δ^9-THC was the only constituent in cannabis which possessed physiological activity. Therefore, it also appeared necessary to design a programme whereby all natural materials and synthetic equivalents could be compared. The state of technical development by this time made it possible to design a national programme, to elucidate a number of basic parameters and to obtain hard core data leading to an understanding of marihuana action. The plan is intended to encourage cooperation in the general research with other investigators throughout the world. The little research that had been accomplished

in the United States before 1966 involved marihuana seized by the
United States Bureau of Narcotics (now the Bureau of Narcotics and
Dangerous Drugs) and furnished to qualified researchers. Unfortunately
much of this material was relatively old, no knowledge about its
potency was available, and the validity of any findings based upon it
is questionable. Researchers must have available materials whose total
chemical constituents and absolute potency are known and identical.
Illicit marihuana is tremendously variable due to age, etc. Seized
materials may be adulterated with other plants and chemical agents,
or may be a mixture of different "varieties" of cannabis.

The synthesis in 1967 by an N.I.M.H. grantee of Δ^9-THC is now
history. The availability of this and related substances, including a
standardized natural product of known potency, will make it possible
to perform the vitally needed pharmacological, biochemical, genetic,
and behavioural research necessary to understand the mode of action
and toxicity of cannabis.

It seems appropriate here to repeat some portions of the history
of this drug, particularly in relation to the United States.

It was cultivated for fibre in the colonies, but its first medical use
in the United States was around 1840 by O'Shaughnessy who had
noted its therapeutic uses while he was stationed in India.

Medical applications rapidly grew, reaching a peak about the time
of World War 1. It was considered therapeutically effective in such
disorders as epilepsy, migraine headache, *anorexia nervosa* and uterine
atony. It was also used as an analgesic and hypnotic. Perhaps difficulties with its standardization and the emergence of new drugs, such
as barbiturates, were factors in its decreased use as a medication.

The description of marihuana use as a vice apparently began in the
State of Louisiana where restrictive laws were passed in 1927. Several
other states followed suit before passage by the United States Government of the Federal Marihuana Tax Law in 1937. Federal narcotic
enforcement officials were active then as now in informing the
American public about a new drug danger, often depicting marihuana
as being more dangerous than the opiates. They requested and received
responsibility for its regulation at the Federal level.

In the thirties and for about twenty five years thereafter marihuana
use was generally confined to minority groups. In 1963, however, there
was a sudden increase in its use by young members of the middle class.
This trend has not diminished but appears to be increasing geometricall·

The medical and scientific communities have a responsibility to define the biological and psychological sequellae of marihuana use in valid public health terms. The National Institute of Mental Health research programme has three phases: (1) Supply; (2) Animal Research; (3) Clinical Research. The objectives of the first two phases are readily understood.

OUTLINE OF PRECLINICAL PROGRAMME ON CANNABIS SATIVA

I. Materials:
    A.   Synthetic Compounds
        1. delta-8-trans-Tetrahydrocannabinol (Δ^8-THC)
        2. delta-9-trans-Tetrahydrocannabinol (Δ^9-THC)
    B.   Marihuana ⎫
        extract   ⎬ crude extract of natural materials
        distillate ⎭
    C.   Plant materials
        1. Free of large stems and seeds
        2. Extracted plant residues
    D.   Radioactive Tagged Compounds
        1. Δ^8-THC ⎫
                  ⎬ — H^3 and C^{14}
        2. Δ^9-THC ⎭

II. Analysis:
    A.   Analytical procedures for control of identity and purity
        1. Δ^8-THC
        2. Δ^9-THC
        3. Other materials in the plant that are active or convertible to active materials
    B.   Analytical methods for qualitative and quantitative determination in tissues of Δ^8-THC and Δ^9-THC
    C.   Stability studies

III. Definition of activities in animals
    A.   Sympathetic system
    B.   Parasympathetic system

C.   Central and peripheral nervous system
D.   Neurotransmitter system

IV. Toxicity
A. LD_{50} of each material
B.   Dose range in
     1. Rats
     2. Dogs
     3. Monkeys
C.   Subacute toxicity (12 weeks)
     1. Rats
     2. Dogs
     3. Monkeys
D.   Chronic toxicity (2 years)
     1. Dogs
     2. Monkeys

V. Biochemical
A.   Absorption
B.   Protein binding
C.   Effects on synthesis, uptake, storage, and release of
     1. Catecholamines
     2. Serotonin
     3. Acetylcholine
     4. Brain circulation
     5. Brain electrolytes—Mg^+, Ca^{++}, K^+, etc.
D.   Drug interactions
     1. MAO inhibitors
     2. Reserpine
     3. Adrenergic blockers (α and β)
     4. Cocaine
     5. Histamine
E.   Examination of specific intracellular particles (amine granules or vesicles)
F.   Metabolism
     1. Active and inactive metabolites
     2. Tolerance and intolerance
     3. Drug dependence

VI. Pyrolysis

    A.   Identification of volatile products from cannabis
    B.   Identification of volatile products from synthetic Δ^8-THC and Δ^9-THC
    C.   Identification of volatile products from nonactive cannabinol-like compounds occurring in the plant, such as cannabinol, cannabidiol, cannabidiolic acid, tetrahydrocannabinolic acid
    D.   Identification of volatile products from extracted plant
    E.   Examination of volatile products from mixture of extracted plant and synthetic Δ^8-THC and Δ^9-THC

In the first six months of the programme, i.e., since July 1968, facilities and experience have become sufficient to grow as much plant material as is needed for the programme in the growing season which is now upon us. Late in 1968, seeds from Turkey, Mexico, Italy (2 "varieties"), France (2 monoecious "varieties"), and Sweden were planted in the State of Mississippi.

Percent Germination of Marihuana Seeds Used in N.I.M.H. Programme— Determined March 1969

(TURKISH)		90%
(FRENCH)	FIBRIMAN 24	14%
(FRENCH)	FIBRIMAN 56	80%
(ITALIAN)	FIBRANOVA	64%
(ITALIAN)	CARMAGNOLA	64%
(SWEDISH)	SVALOF 60703	18%

Wild collections were also made in various parts of the United States. Data is being collected on the Δ^9-THC content of these plant materials.

Alternative procedures for extracting the plant materials have been tried. A large batch of material confiscated by the Bureau of Narcotics and furnished to the programme, containing 1.312% Δ^9-THC, was extracted with alcohol, concentrated to a low volume, diluted with water, and extracted with hexane. The hexane extracted material was then distilled in a molecular still. The first batch of the resulting oily material, the "marihuana extract distillate", contains about 20% of Δ^9-THC; 2% cannabidiol; 6.4% cannabinol; and more than 50% of a terpene-like material. Analysis by gas chromatography at critical points during the processing indicated that the cannabinoid constituents were not altered, either as to character or as to their ratio of occurrence. Since it is not known what effects, if any, terpene-like materials will have on the active constituents and their absorption, it was decided that this product should be used as the basic plant extract to be compared with synthetic materials. Further fractionation of the hexane extracted material and products therefrom will be examined for physiological activity and toxicity. The work done on this material from an unknown source will determine the procedure for processing the "homegrown" marihuana.

Reference standards of Δ^8-THC have been produced by synthesis. Reference samples of other cannabinoid compounds will be produced either by synthesis or obtained from the plant extracts.

We would welcome information on sources of supply of any of the cannabinoids, as well as about additional cannabinoids which may be isolated and identified in the future.

Synthesis of 2½ Kg of Δ^8-THC is complete. Some tritiated Δ^8-THC has been made, and additional quantities will be prepared and made available for certain crucial experiments. At least 80% of the tritium atom is in the 8-position in the Δ^8-THC, the balance being on the 9-methyl, the 10-position and the aromatic ring. C^{14} will be randomly distributed in the aromatic ring of the tetrahydrocannabinols.

Large quantities of Δ^9-THC can also be prepared. As soon as intermediates can be accumulated, a pilot plant batch of about 2½ Kg will be produced.

Work on the identification of pyrolytic products in smoking experiments has been started.

Gas chromatographic analysis has been developed to a high degree within each of the laboratories involved in the work (see list at end of this paper). New methods of determining cannabinoids and their metabolic products in body fluids and tissues are being sought.

The major portion of research in the programme to date has been by contract, but some research is supported by grants.

The Centre for Studies of Narcotic and Drug Abuse reviews drug abuse grant applications. Previously, grant applications for the study of both abuse and therapeutic uses of marihuana were directed to the Psychopharmacology Research Branch of N.I.M.H. The present interest of that Branch is research into therapeutic applications of analogues of components from cannabis. Examples of the kinds of work which have been or are supported currently by it include:

(a) to study the metabolic transformation which THC undergoes "in vivo"; a study in animals utilizing tritium labelled Δ^8-THC;

(b) to study the chemical constituents of marihuana; to synthesize them and to study their psychopharmacological activity;

(c) to analyse C^{14}-marihuana by TLC, to separate and isolate working quantities of C^{14}-tagged cannabinoids;

(d) to improve metabolic studies;

(e) to examine the effects of marihuana preparations and synthetic cannabinols, administered repeatedly before or during gestation, on the mammalian reproductive processes. Possible effects of interest: altered fertility of either sex, failure of normal prenatal and postnatal development or reduced viability of the offspring; altered neurological or behavioural characteristics of the offspring; effect on various aspects of reproduction through as many as four successive generations;

(f) to study the effects of two active marihuana principles on the CNS, the cardiovascular system and on the biochemical interactions with various enzyme systems and biogenic amines; effects on spontaneous motor activity, interaction with reserpine and barbiturates, tests for amphetamine-like properties and a battery of behavioural procedures, etc.

MECHANISM FOR DISTRIBUTION OF CANNABIS AND CANNABIS CONSTITUENTS BY THE NATIONAL INSTITUTE OF MENTAL HEALTH

The N.I.M.H., which is the research arm of the United States Government dealing with C.N.S. agents, was chosen (after consultation with the Bureau of Narcotics and Dangerous Drugs and the Food and Drug Administration) to control and distribute marihuana and its constituents.

United States scientists apply to the National Institute of Mental Health for supplies. Details are available on request. The researcher furnishes documents which attest to his qualifications. The Bureau of Narcotics and Dangerous Drugs determines the legitimacy of the application. The scientific review is accomplished by an advisory committee responsible to the Director, National Institute of Mental Health. The members of this committee have conducted extensive investigations with cannabis and are considered experts in the field.

After review of the protocol, the request may be approved, approved with advice to improve the research design, deferred with communication, or disapproved. Since supplies of material are in short supply, priorities are determined on the basis of merit or scientific value, quality and kind of data expected. Disapprovals generally result when the study does not fit in with the time-table or specific objectives of the programme.

The requirements for human studies of the U.S. Food and Drug Administration must be satisfied and evidence of this must be furnished to the N.I.M.H. when the research is to be conducted in man.

Regarding human studies, the marihuana committee, which also advises the Institute of research which should be supported, has described the conditions under which cannabis and its constituents can be used safely in clinical research with humans. The following criteria apply:

(1) evidence of the approval of the appropriate institutional committee on human studies shall be provided;
(2) the number of subjects shall be stated or estimated;
(3) physical, psychiatric and physiological screening of subject(s) shall be conducted;
(4) the institutional setting and safeguards against adverse reactions and for handling patients during the post-drug period shall be stated;
(5) the number of times a given subject may be exposed to the drug shall be stated.

To date, very limited quantities of marihuana plant material have been provided to researchers other than to the contractors supported by the N.I.M.H. for the basic studies. The material furnished, described earlier, has been used almost exclusively for pilot experiments on research planned for the future.

The published effects of marihuana appear to suggest that the area of research which should now be evaluated critically in humans should not be too circumscribed.

We do not know enough about the long-term effects of marihuana use. As in the case of tobacco, it is possible that there are serious consequences of chronic use which will become apparent only through careful and longitudinal studies. Neither must we forget the need of therapy for the adverse effects of marihuana. We therefore have an intense interest in finding and developing an antidote for cannabis intoxication.

We are not pursuing the social, psychological and medical aspects in depth at this time, but this must be undertaken very soon.

List of contracts from N.I.M.H.

The Research Institute of Pharmaceutical Sciences, School of Pharmacy, University of Mississippi, will grow at least five varieties of marihuana. It will provide a supply of natural material with a fully defined history and analysis. This natural material will also be used for comparison with synthetic THC.

The Research Triangle Institute, Durham, North Carolina (three contracts), will extract marihuana supplied to it by the Bureau of Narcotics and Dangerous Drugs. Purification procedures will be developed and specified materials will be provided to N.I.M.H. Some synthetic THC will be tagged with radioactive atoms.

Arthur D. Little, Inc. Cambridge, Massachusetts (two contracts), will test methods for producing THC and will prepare large quantities of synthetic THC.

The Battelle Memorial Institute, Columbus, Ohio, will analyse marihuana smoke and its constituents and will attempt to determine which of these compounds are absorbed into the user's system.

The N.I.M.H. contracts for these programmes total $419,057.

DISCUSSION 3: PHARMACOLOGICAL ASPECTS

Schultes   I think it would be very interesting from the chemical and botanical points of view to compare the yellow-brown, burnt-looking leaves from the Mexican plant with normal leaves. It could be a faulty potassium metabolism in one part of the plant. It could be many other things, but this happens with a number of cultivated plants, and it would be very interesting to see whether this could affect the bio-synthesis of the interesting compounds.

Crombie   I would suggest that cannabigerol, cannabicyclol and cannabichromene be added to the N.I.M.H. list of synthetic compounds. The problem of solubility, which Prof. Paton mentioned, is very important. We thought of making the tetrahydrocannabinol and the extracts in oil, for oral application. We have given it in olive oil, for example, for subcutaneous injection.

Mechoulam   Can you not give it by intravenous injections, anyway?

Bein   You still have to dilute it. You can. We have given it intra-venously to cats, dogs and rats.

Mechoulam   I have heard that polyethylene glycol 400 is a very good solubilizing agent.

Fairbairn   I asked a physical chemist if one could form a complex with phosphonitrate. He thought this compound would be very suitable.

Paton   I think it would be quite easy to get some sort of a complex, but what happens in the animal? Where would the complex be carried, and where will it break down? At the moment I am backing Tween 80 which unfortunately releases histamine.

Joyce   Four years ago, Prof. Bergl suggested that dimethylsulphoxide might be worth trying. This also has some tiresome pharmacology of its own, but it is a very good vehicle for many purposes. Has it been tried for THC?

Miras   Dimethylsulphoxide is an excellent solvent, but the distribution of THC is then quite different as you can find with autoradiographs. We have also tried to introduce THC by mixing it with serum from the animal, but the pharmacological activity and the distribution is still slightly different.

Joyce   It is conceivable that the distribution with DMSO or with some other solvent might resemble the distribution after normal smoking, rather than intravenous administration. The fact that distribution depends upon the solvent is no disqualification in itself.

Petrzilka   The actual pattern of distribution resembles that found with LSD; a very low concentration in the brain, a lot in the small intestines, little in the blood and so forth.

A. S. Curry   And high concentration in the lungs.

Paton   What really matters is the concentration in the basal parts of the brain, and this is seldom known.

Do I gather that both Dr. Agurell and Prof. Mechoulam do not find THC as such in the urine, nor cannabinol? Prof. Korte said he thought it was coming out in the urine.

Mechoulam   Our metabolite under hydrolytic conditions will turn into cannabinol, first by chopping off the conjugate and then by dehydration.

Paton   To determine how much cannabis, or whether any has been taken, obviously it is going to be very difficult to break the conjugation and convert it into cannabinol.

Mechoulam   I had hoped that by isolating it immediately one would not have to estimate such small amounts as is necessary at present.

Curry   I think this is the way we have got to go. Until we have the authentic metabolite crystallized and characterized, we have to turn the metabolite into something that we can identify.

Miras   I should say that we have not found much difference between our experience during the past four years with humans and the work of Dr. Agurell on animals. The small differences are probably due to the routes of administration. In humans the lungs very quickly get a lot of the radioactivity after smoking; a lot of the THC, given by intraperitoneal injection is, of course, only absorbed much later. A lot of different compounds are present after smoking THC. Most are in combined form: only a little is free. After two days there is still some radioactivity in the urine.

We have asked our police contacts to mix radioactive material (labelled with Iodine[131]) with the other and then to follow the resulting "traffic". We were able to pick up a lot of people who smoked this labelled compound, and from them I was able to collect a lot of urine and from some the bile as well. After six hours there was quite a lot of radioactivity in the bile, as was the case in experiments on rat bile that we have already published.

The people who collect the material from the fields for me are often affected by absorbing the material in some way—they get headaches, dizziness, sleepiness, and they go to sleep much earlier and they have other reactions. Hashish smokers I have known for twenty years are now able to smoke at least ten times as much as other people. If a beginner smoked the same quantity he would collapse. Incidentally, if collapse from hashish smoking does need treatment, what they get is lemon juice.

Shulgin   How is the iodine fixed to the hashish? Is it elemental iodine?

Miras   Yes.
Crombie   Do you iodinate the phenol?
Miras   Yes. The action is as good, or even stronger in fact. Perhaps
the mobility of the material is changed.
Shulgin   This is a gross amount of iodination. It implies that you are
generating a trace amount of an extraordinarily active material, with
a different pharmacology.
Miras   You have to reduce the dose by one-third.
Mechoulam   I am unaware of a generally accepted antidote for
Cannabis. Kudrin and Davydova (1968) used phenitrone. Grunfeld and

Phenitrone

Edery (1969) have reported that amphetamine reversed the behavioural
changes elicited by Δ^1-THC in monkeys. Burroughs (1966) reports that
apomorphine promptly relieves anxiety caused by Cannabis.
Bein   Last year, we received a petroleum-ether extract of cannabis
containing 24% THC, and, in addition, pure THC from Professor
Korte. We tested the preparations in mice, rats, rabbits, cats and dogs.
When I say "we", I mean a group of friends and co-workers: the
pharmacologists Dr. Jaques, Dr. Pericin and Dr. Helfer, and the biochemists Dr. Staehelin and Dr. Maître.

   I do not wish to go into details, but I should like to mention some
of our findings. Psychopharmacological agents other than THC have
certain effects in common: for instance, they regularly give rise to a
decrease in motility, catatonia, a decrease in body temperature, and
tranquillization that is sometimes interrupted by periods of increased
excitability. With the THC preparations, we were not able to detect
any activity that could have been described as hallucinogenic, although
we did observe certain reactions that might perhaps have been
interpreted as signs of such a pharmacological property.

   Like many well-known psychopharmacological agents, reserpine,
chlorpromazine, and, to a lesser extent, imipramine, the THC preparations antagonized the increase in motor activity induced by
mescaline in the mouse instead of the synergism that might have been
expected.

   Now reserpine, imipramine, and chlorpromazine influence the
endogenous catecholamines, each of these three agents acting in quite

a characteristic manner. The THC preparations did not exert any
reserpine-like activity on the catecholamines; furthermore, we did not
observe any inhibition of the uptake of noradrenaline in the rat
heart—a phenomenon that is very typical of imipramine; on the
contrary, the uptake of noradrenaline tended to increase. These
experiments were carried out with tritium-labelled noradrenaline. THC
therefore, had no imipramine-like activity, at least with regard to
catecholamine metabolism. This was further substantiated by the
fact that in the tetrabenazine-test THC displayed no antagonistic
activity (such as is found with imipramine) but a synergistic one.

On the other hand, THC did influence the catecholamines in the
brain, inasmuch as it activated tyrosine-hydroxylase; this may be
regarded as an indication that THC increases the biosynthesis of
catecholamines in the brain. (The animals received tritium-labelled
tyrosine in our experiments; the tritium-labelled catecholamines—
and hence the transformation of tyrosine into catecholamines—were
determined.) Activation of tyrosine-hydroxylase was first described
in connection with chlorpromazine. According to Levitt, Spector,
Sjoerdsma and Udenfriend, tyrosine-hydroxylase is the rate-limiting
step in the biosynthesis of noradrenaline.

Before we can draw any conclusions with regard to the relevance
of these findings in relation to clinical observations in man and
results in the animal, we shall have to elaborate on them and test
other chemical fractions and constituents of cannabis; it looks to
me, however, as if this might be an interesting approach.

Joyce   One theme that has come up two or three times is whether it
it better to work from synthetic materials or to make extracts. Clearly
the answer will depend to some extent upon the circumstances. Has
the time now come when, in order to work out the animal, let alone
the human pharmacology, it might be preferable to get all extracts
from a standard source, such as the N.I.M.H. programme, rather than
to prepare one's own? Clearly, irrelevant but misleading differences
are possible otherwise. To what extent is it possible for people outside
the United States to obtain materials from N.I.M.H.? There are
rumours that N.I.M.H. is already saturated with demands for these
materials that they are unable to meet.

Scigliano   We have established two sources of supply: one for research
in my area, and one for forensic use within the Bureau of Narcotics. At
this moment our supplies are rather limited, but we evaluate the request
on the basis of how it fits into the programme that I have described.

Joyce   It might well be convenient if N.I.M.H. and the Bureau of
Narcotics were not the only source.

Mechoulam We have been supplying quite a few people: the police,
N.I.M.H., the Narcotics Bureau in the United States. We do not want
to turn into a factory producing THC, and there is now a firm willing
to do it. They will be able to supply research people who can send an
official document from their government that they are allowed to
import the material.

Braenden The United Nations Laboratory would be prepared to
undertake the distribution of such material placed at its disposal. One
of the functions of the U.N. Laboratory has been the provision of
basic research material to scientists. During the past 10 years, the
Laboratory has sent many cannabis samples to its collaborators. Such
an arrangement enables different investigators to carry out research
on the same samples, and so to compare the results obtained. Previously,
such comparisons were not possible. I would also like to draw attention
to the United Nations ST/SOA/SER.S/.. series of documents which is
devoted to scientific research on cannabis. The publication of papers
in this series has several advantages. There is very little delay between
the submission of a document and its publication and there is a very
wide distribution, both in English and French, to scientists carrying
out research on cannabis. We have especially tried to emphasize in this
series the importance of publishing negative as well as positive results
in order to minimize duplication of effort. Finally, I would like to
mention the important collection of scientific literature on narcotic
drugs at the United Nations Laboratory in Geneva and the system
which has been developed there for the rapid retrieval of information.
I invite those of you who may be in Geneva in the future to visit us at
the Laboratory and to consult the literature there.

Joyce I would like to testify personally to the excellence of
Dr. Braenden's literature collection. Can I ask everybody here, their
friends and colleagues and eventual readers of the Proceedings, to form
the habit of sending any information that they have collected to the
Institute for the Study of Drug Dependence as well as to Dr. Braenden,
even before publication? Of course it can be subject to any restrictions
on further communication they wish to put upon it. We would like
to be sure that this is one way in which we continue and extend this
collaboration that we have begun with you.

References

Burroughs, W. S., in *The Marihuana Papers,* Ed. D. Solomon, The
        Bobbs-Merill Co. Inc., New York, 1966, pp. 392-3.

Grunfeld, Y. and Edery, H., *Psychopharmacologia* (*Berl.*), 14:200
        (1969).

Kudrin, A. N. and Davydova, N. O., *Farmakologiya: Toksikologiya*
        549 (1968).

APPENDIX

NOMENCLATURE

Numbering Systems, Formulae, Trivial Names and Suggested Abbreviations for Various Cannabinoids

L. Crombie

Numbering Systems

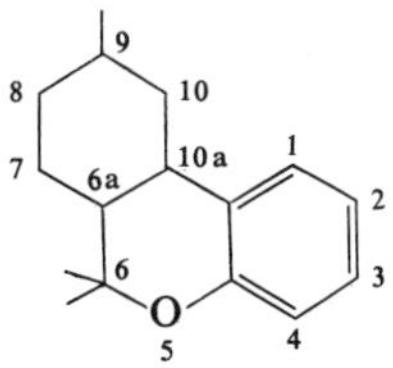

I
Dibenzopyran
numbering

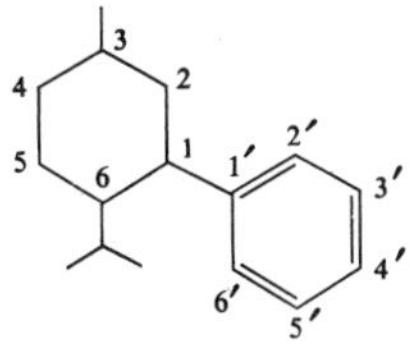

II
Biphenyl
numbering

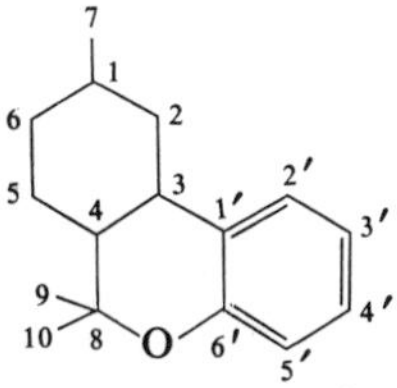

III
Monoterpenoid
numbering

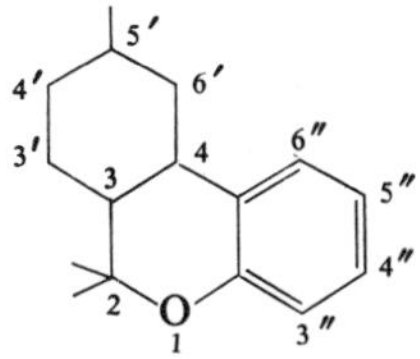

IV
Earlier, Chemical Society
(London), numbering

Notes: The dibenzopyran numbering is used by Chemical Abstracts and is sometimes employed in conjunction with biphenyl numbering, the latter for cannabidiol types, etc. A number of authors prefer the monoterpenoid numbering which is used for tetrahydrocannabinol and cannabidiol types alike. The Chemical Society numbering was used on older papers.

209

Some Important Hashish Extractives (True Natural Products or Artefacts)*

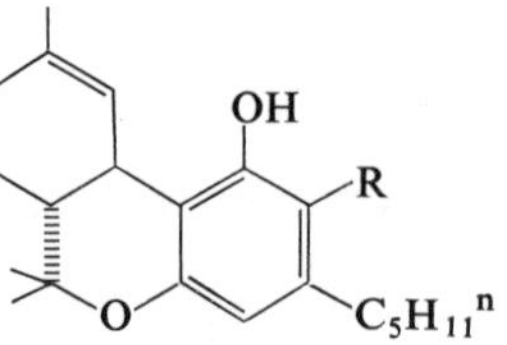

V

R = H: Δ^1-Tetrahydrocannabinol (Δ^1-THC)[a,b], or
Δ^9-Tetrahydrocannabinol (Δ^9-THC)
R = CO_2H: Δ^1-Tetrahydrocannabinolic acid (Δ^1-THCA), or
Δ^9-Tetrahydrocannabinolic acid (Δ^9-THCA).

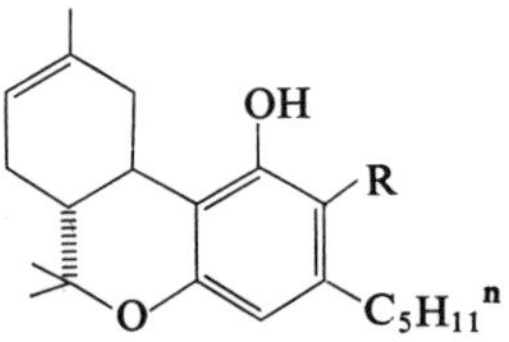

VI

R = H: $\Delta^{1,(6)}$-Tetrahydrocannabinol ($\Delta^{1,(6)}$-THC)[a,b], or
$\Delta^{6,1}$-Tetrahydrocannabinol ($\Delta^{6,1}$-THC), or
Δ^8-Tetrahydrocannabinol (Δ^8-THC)
R = CO_2H: $\Delta^{1,(6)}$-Tetrahydrocannabinolic acid ($\Delta^{1,(6)}$-THCA), or
$\Delta^{6,1}$-Tetrahydrocannabinolic acid ($\Delta^{6,1}$-THCA), or
Δ^8-Tetrahydrocannabinolic acid (Δ^8-THCA).

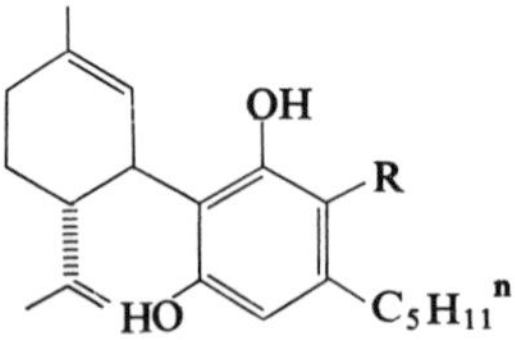

VII

R = H: Cannabidiol (CD)[b]
R = CO_2H: Cannabidiolic acid (CDA)

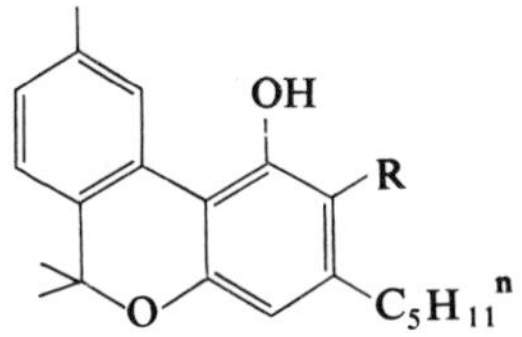

VIII
R = H: Cannabinol (CN).
R = CO_2H: Cannabinolic acid (CNA).

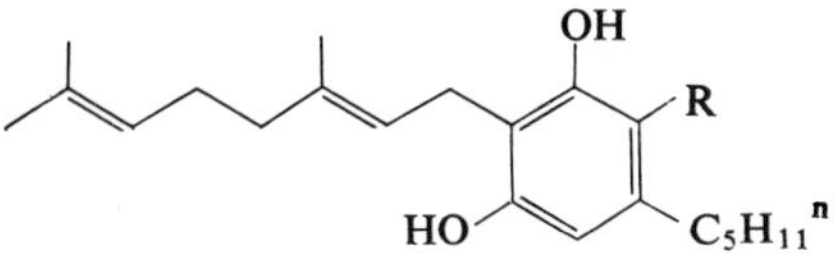

IX
R = H: Cannabigerol (CG)
R = CO_2H: Cannabigerolic acid (CGA).

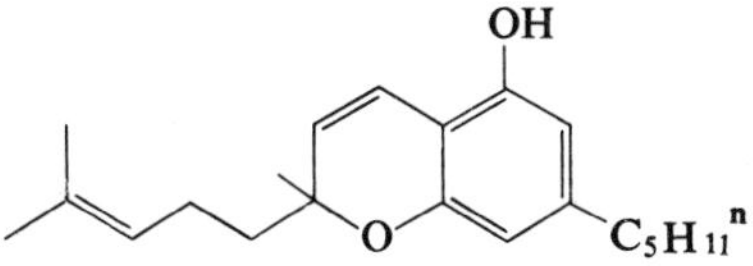

X
Cannabichromene (CC)[c]

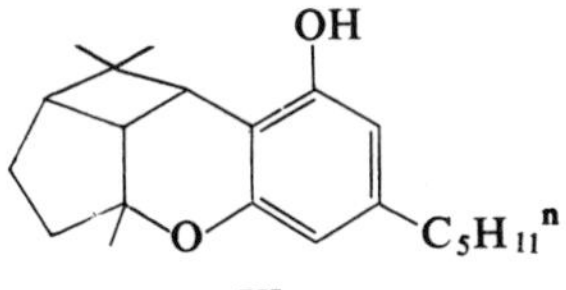

XI
Cannabicyclol (CCY)[c]

Notes: [a] *trans*-Fused from natural sources.
[b] Absolute stereochemistry established as shown.
[c] Apparently optically inactive, as obtained from hashish.

Relevant Synthetic Structures*

XII

3,4-*cis*-Δ^1-Tetrahydrocannabinol (Δ^1-*cis*-THC), or
6a,10a-*cis*-Δ^9-Tetrahydrocannabinol (Δ^9-*cis*-THC)

XIII   XIV

$\Delta^{8,(9)}$-Isotetrahydrocannabinol ($\Delta^{8,(9)}$-IsoTHC)

XV   XVI

Citrylidene-cannabis (CIC)

Note: *Suggested abbreviations follow each name, in parentheses.

Subject Index

Entries in italics indicate the first entry in a section of text particularly concerned with the subject indicated.

213